Keto Fasting Mastery

Follow the Ultimate Complete Guide for Burning Fat Off Your Body, by Transitioning to a Low Carbohydrate/ Ketogenic Diet Whilst Fasting for Men and Women!

By Georgia Bolton

"Keto and Intermittent Fasting Mastery: Follow the Ultimate Complete Guide for Burning Fat Off Your Body, by Transitioning to a Low Carbohydrate/ Ketogenic Diet Whilst Fasting for Men and Women!" Written by "Georgia Bolton".

Keto and Intermittent Fasting Mastery is a bundle of the books "Keto Mastery", & "Intermittent Fasting Mastery".

Hope You Enjoy!

Keto Mastery

Follow the Advanced Ketogenic/ Low Carbohydrate Diet That Many Top Performing Men and Women Athletes Have Used for Reaching Peak Performance By Following This Complete Dieting Guide!

By Georgia Bolton

Table of Contents

3. Ketosis is free reign to stuff your craw with deep-fried butter and pork belly

4. Nutrient proportions are set in stone

5. Ketosis is a risk factor for ketoacidosis

6. Ketosis is the ultimate, final way to lose weight

7. Ketosis is a high protein diet

8. Ketosis destroys your heart and valves

9. Keto can cause flu-like symptoms

10. Ketosis exacerbates fatty liver

11. Ketosis carries out a systematic extermination of your gut flora

12. Any fat is good fat

And so it is written

Chapter 11: Good Foods

Fats and oils

Meat, poultry, and seafood

Nuts, Seeds, Legumes, etc.:

Fruits:

Vegetables:

Dairy

Snacks:

Drinks:

Foods to avoid, or at least eat in moderation:

Fats:

Meats:

Starches

Fruits

Vegetables

Sugars, sweeteners, desserts, etc.

Snacks

Drinks:

Conclusion

Table of Contents

Introduction

The public consciousness is bubbling with all manner of diets and weight loss strategies - from intermittent fasting to the Atkins diet to the Paleo diet. The one that seems to be continuously mysterious to a lot of people is the ketogenic diet, or keto, for short. Is it a high protein, high fat diet? Low carb diet? Neither of these - the keto diet is based on the principle of changing the body from a carbohydrate-powered metabolic engine to a fat-powered one. The name "ketogenic" comes from the compounds that are the end result of the breakdown of fatty acids in the liver when there is not enough sugar in the bloodstream, called ketones. When blood glucose is low, either via fasting or by a particular diet, the body breaks down stored fat into ketones as fuel.

Now how does all this apply to the diet? Essentially, the ketogenic diet is one that revolves around the high-fat intake, moderate protein intake, and very low-carbohydrate intake to keep your body in a state of "ketosis" - burning ketones for fuel instead of sugar.

Interestingly, the genesis of the ketogenic diet lies in the treatment of epilepsy. Treatises from ancient Greece going back as far as 400 BCE prescribe the use of fasting to treat seizures. Obviously, they didn't know it, but fasting bodies created ketones to fuel themselves. In the early 20th century, Rollin Turner Woodyatt used it to treat epileptic patients with some success. In the 1990s, it received national attention again as a treatment for epilepsy, and from there, the diet gained momentum and other similar diets emerged such as the Atkins diet and Paleo diet.

How do the keto, Atkins, and the paleo diet differ from each other, you may ask? If you look into a nutrition magazine, you'll be up to your eyeballs with those three and a thousand more strategies.

To keep it concise, keto and Atkins are fairly similar. The primary difference is that the goal of Keto is to put you in ketosis, a metabolic state of burning ketones for fuel, while Atkins is centered around strictly weight loss. Atkins also is more structured in its approach, classically containing four different "stages" and which are based around time and amount of weight lost. Finally, and most notably, the Atkins diet is more generous in its carbohydrate consumption.

The paleo diet revolves around trying to recreate a hypothetical "caveman" diet of unprocessed foods, composed primarily of organic protein and vegetables. What's more important to the paleo diet is the particular food choices, not necessarily a delicate balance of fat, protein, and carbohydrates.

The paleo diet has a lot in common with other diets, in that it emphasizes whole food choices over processed ones, and usually ethically-sourced ones at that, but does not really concern itself with macronutrient balance and ketosis.

Ketosis is a big subject, with many facets to consider, from how it fixes the modern diet to what to eat. If you're interested in changing your energy systems, read on. The knowledge in this book should put you on the path to a more informed and healthier version of yourself.

Chapter 1: The Problems with the Modern Diet

As many people are probably already aware, we are in the midst of something that can be described aptly as a global metabolic crisis. Obesity, heart disease, and type-2 diabetes rates are higher than ever before and still climbing, not only in the developed world but even in burgeoning countries. The reason for this is simply too massive a topic to be covered in this book, but what it comes down is nutritional havoc perpetrated by excessive simple carbohydrate consumption. When you eat simple carbs, they are easily broken down by body into their component sugars, which causes the pancreas to release insulin, which stores some of those component sugars as glycogen in the muscle and liver, to be used as immediate, quick-to-access energy, and the rest to be deposited in our fat cells, making us to balloon up. In addition, they amongst the easiest to acquire and rewarding foods known to man, being cheap, widely available, and versatile. Simple carbohydrates cover a range from the more commonly known choices like candy and doughnuts, typically what someone thinks of when they hear "simple" or "bad" carbs, to daily staples like bread, rice, and pasta.

Theoretically, if one entered a prolonged state of carb withdrawal, a fast or diet composed primarily of fat and protein, your body does what it naturally does - consumes the stored carbohydrates in your body, the glycogen in your muscles and liver, for energy and then starts tapping into the fat cells for sustenance - ketosis. The problem is, our modern world, we never get to this point. Our world is one where food is widely available, and the quickest, cheapest, easiest, and most rewarding things to eat are carbohydrates, forestalling your ketogenic state forever unless one makes the conscious and informed choice to enter it.

One of the problems is in the United States especially, for most of the 20th century, there was a strong backlash against dietary fat based on faulty science that started long, destructive love affair with carbohydrates that we're still collectively getting over. The term "fat" to refer to lipids was probably one of the worst things PR wise that could have happened to them, as the association was obvious - fat makes you fat. That's the most natural conclusion in the world to make, right? Well, human metabolism is never that simple, and the maxim of "fat is the enemy" has been simply destructive on our collective health. Carbohydrates are also inherently less filling than fats, meaning one has to consume more of them to attain the same satiety that fat does. It's true that fat has a higher calorie per gram count, nine per gram, about double carbohydrate's four per gram, so satiety one feels is much greater, usually leading one to consume fewer calories at the end of the day. That's another advantage of the keto diet; you'll be feeling so satisfied from your diet that there's no longer a need to accidentally consume 400 calories in chips or other snacks.

With that in mind, ever looked at the calorie count on a can of soda or a glass of fruit juice? They're almost always in excess of 100, all packed it into a neat little can or bottle and does nothing for actual feelings of hunger, and these products are EVERYWHERE. In the case of fruit juice, it's being marketed as healthy even though almost all the things that keep fruit from being a metabolic insulin bomb have been stripped away.

Despite the huge prevalence of these sorts of foods everywhere, the idea of "fat is the enemy" still has a decent amount of weight behind it (no pun intended); think about how many products you see marketing themselves as healthier and better for you for being low in fat - in reality, if you want to send your body's fat-burning systems into overdrive, consuming fat and avoiding carbs is the headspace you want to be in.

Unfortunately, today we live in a fast-paced world where convenience is king and the quicker something can be done, the better. This has led to an increase in processed foods, foods artificially preserved with harmful chemicals and stripped of all base nutritional content in the process. In fact, with a lot of foods, including white flour, white rice, and pasta, nutrients have to be added back in to make sure that people don't suffer from certain deficiencies that would be easy to avoid in a world of whole foods. The other unfortunate reality is that almost every single processed food is packed to the brim with sugar, and in the case of things like pastries, are also made of insulin spiking white flour.

Processed foods high in oil always take the cheapest possible way out, with oil that's cheap to produce and heavily processed in of itself, usually a saturated fat or, even worse, trans fats. Trans fats are hydrogenated vegetable fats and are easy to store for a long time and melt at temperatures considered desirable, and are commonly used in things like mass-produced pastries and fast food.

What does hydrogenated mean? To properly get ahold of this, one needs to understand the chemical structure of fats. Fats have long chains of bonded hydrogen and carbon when bonded together once, they're called saturated, and twice, they're called unsaturated. Hydrogenation is simply the process of changing an unsaturated (liquid at room temperature, canola, peanut, or corn oil) fat to a saturated (Solid at room temperature, think butter, lard, or coconut oil) one by changing the chemical bonds of carbon from double to single. What are the ramifications of all these chemical shenanigans for your body? They end up increasing the amount of "bad" cholesterol, LDLs and drop the amount of "good" cholesterol, HDLs, increase triglycerides in blood, and increase inflammation all around the body. These sorts of oils are found nearly everywhere, in almost every processed and fast food, and, as mentioned before, convenience is king. People are on the run, people are busy, and are more interested in temporarily squashing hunger pangs than the long-term implications of their diet and food choices. Instead of fixing a simple and filling meal at home that is high in protein and healthy fats, people are opting for the simpler choice.

How to Fix It

What can be done to remedy the modern diet? The good thing about today's world is that healthy food is cheaper than ever, and the internet acts as a veritable infinite library of information for every food under the sun, and the ones still buried. It just takes a trained eye and a mind well trained in proper decisions about "whole" foods. For the sake of this book, take whole foods to mean unprocessed meats, wild seafood, raw dairy, fresh fruit and vegetables, dried beans, and minimally processed, whole grains.

Following the keto diet isn't a prerequisite for health, but mindfulness about your food choices is, and that's where everyone should start. To start assessing how badly the modern diet has blown out your body, a mental note should be made of what you eat and be diligent to change what needs to be changed. It's not a simple process - renovating any part of your life is never easy - but the simplest place to start is possibly in identifying any food choices that stick out to you as bad. We all know the ones that claw at the back of our minds – the guilty pleasures, the "convenience" foods, the elaborate coffees that are basically desserts that we're all so fond of, things you know it would be best for you to cut out. That's where this book starts, just trying to get you to be more cognizant of what you eat, to take the first step and eliminate some of the choices that you know are bad for you, the foods that are helping you to pack on an extra layer of fluff for winter, despite the fact that there's a good chance you won't be spending it in a cave. Once that first step is taken, the rest can follow suit so much easier.

Setting goals is always a good idea, be it financially, professionally, personally, or fitness wise. Goals give you a sense of illuminating purpose, and, in a way, light a path for you to follow along to your destination. Start small and get bigger – is your goal to eat more fiber, protein, to put on healthy weight, or to lose bad weight? Once you have a goal in mind, more serious planning can occur. You base your food choices around what you want to mold your body into.

Getting Informed

To properly fix the train wreck that is the modern diet, one needs to know how exactly to implement healthier choices. This is a neglected aspect of modern education for many people, despite how absolutely essential to health and happiness it is. We live in an age where there is more information freely circulating about any topic you can imagine, yet for some reason, this information has failed to properly diffuse across the modern consciousness. It's no wonder that in an age where processed, artificially crafted foods are so common and cheap, people, in their woeful ignorance, are forsaking actual healthy choices, which is causing diabetes, obesity and heart disease to run rampant.

To get a basic gestalt of the different nutrients, a short guide will be provided here:

- Carbohydrates: Energy, the most bioavailable fuel source. Made up of sugars; bread, pasta, rice, beans, starchy vegetables, and other grains
- Fat/Lipids: Stored energy of plants and animals, made of a glycerin molecule with fatty acids attached. High satiety. Vegetable oils, butter, lard.
- Proteins: Structural component of living tissue, helps maintain and build tissues. Composed of amino acids. Meat, fish, eggs, dairy products, and tofu.
- Fiber: Indigestible carbohydrate necessary for gut health, keeps hunger and blood sugar in check. Found in unprocessed whole grains (Whole wheat pasta, bread, brown rice) beans, fruits, and vegetables
- Vitamins and Minerals: Two distinct micronutrients, meaning they're needed in small amounts, for various body functions such as muscle action, digestion, eye health, and dozens of other roles.

This brings us nicely into the next point; fiber is *extremely* important for satiety and keeping blood sugar stable. Sudden spikes in blood sugar cause it to be stored as fat by insulin and the feared "sugar crash," getting sleepy after polishing off a plate of pasta or bowl of rice.

Simple Versus Complex Carbohydrates

This is probably a term you've heard before, but doubtless, the true meaning is somewhere floating in a metaphorical miasma around your (and millions of other's) minds. Simple carbs are easily broken down by the body and spike the blood sugar. That fact was touched on earlier in this chapter, but it neglected to define a complex carb. Complex carbs are not as refined as simple ones, they don't have their fiber, and nutritious bits stripped away, and because of that, they are harder for your body to break down, don't spike your blood sugar and cause you to feel full longer. If one desires to be healthier, complex is the way to go.

They keep cravings off and keep your belly feeling full and happy for hours after, as well as maintaining their micronutrient profile of vitamins and minerals. The USDA recommended fiber intake for adults is between 20 and 30, and that's easy to get when your diet is filled with things like vegetables, fruit, whole grain bread, pasta, brown rice, and beans. Common knowledge also dictates that vegetables are absolutely essential for health for other reasons, they are full of antioxidants and are among the most micronutrient dense foods on earth, not counting chunks of animals some would consider rather unpalatable, namely liver, kidneys, sweetbreads, and the like.

Fats and Proteins

While fiber is important for satiety, your body can't run off it. Fat helps keep you fueled, and if you get it from healthy animal sources, grass-fed beef and butter, heritage pigs, and monounsaturated oils like olive oil, coconut oil, and avocado, there's nothing to be feared in terms of hidden health dangers. Protein is also essential for maintaining your living tissue, keeping your hundreds of muscles and organs maintained and strong.

In times of ketosis, whether via fasting or conscious decision, protein is broken via gluconeogenesis (Gluco = sugar, Neo = New, Genesis = Creation) to fuel the brain, as well as being used to maintain body composition, and keeping you full. This makes protein something you can't afford to neglect, keto diet or not.

Fats come in a few different ~~flavors~~ *Types* – monounsaturated, polyunsaturated, trans, and saturated. Monounsaturated are your "good fats," liquid at room temperature fats like olive, almond, and avocado oil, and are composed of numerous heart-healthy fatty acids and usually have other micronutrients as well. Polyunsaturated are not as good for you, but not necessarily bad, corn, canola, soybean oil. They can still be good for the body, but not as much as their monounsaturated brothers. Trans fats are to be avoided at all costs due to a serious link with heart disease. The most mysterious sibling of the fat family is saturated fat, solid at room temperature. Animal fats and coconut oil – depending on the quality of the source (Happier animals or virgin coconut oil) saturated fat can have serious health benefits, from hormone regulation to omega-3s, but it might impact your blood lipid levels, depending on genes, diet, and activity levels. Don't cut it out altogether, but try not to make dinner lard with a side of coconut oil.

Putting it all Together

Now that the information has been passed to you, it's relatively easy to start putting a diet together to remedy the many problems of the modern diet. While a ketogenic diet is going to be the main focus of the rest of this book, it can be hard for a lot of people to go full keto, and the point of this chapter was more to elucidate you on basic diet choices. A healthy panacea to the modern dietary disaster would be a diet with little to no simple carbohydrates, only coming from fruit if possible, high in complex carbs in the form of vegetables and whole grains and beans. The rest should be built from healthy, sustainable proteins and fats to keep you full, happy, and functional. Buying expensive organic products isn't necessary, and oftentimes they aren't necessarily better for you, just containing a slightly different micronutrient profile. What's more important for your immediate health is keeping a good macronutrient profile rich in fiber, vitamins, and minerals.

Chapter 2: The Good Parts of Keto

Keto has been espoused across by people in all walks of life as a powerful tool to lose weight, improve athletic performance, reduce brain fog, control cravings and increase self-control, lower insulin resistance, control certain diseases, and even save money and time.

Keto and Weight Loss

To learn how the ketogenic diet helps you lose weight, one must first visualize how the body stores its excess energy – as fat. All the fat on the human body, or adipose tissue, represents a huge reservoir of potential energy, that could last us up to weeks. What happens with a lot of people is that that fat never really gets tapped in to, as the continuous flow of carbs into the body defeats the need for the body to break into its supply. When you starve your body of carbohydrates, it turns to its stored fat for fuel, a state of ketosis, producing ketones. Ketones are like the backup generator for your body, produced in the liver, and triggered by low blood sugar. Lipase, an enzyme, cleaves off some of the stored triglycerides, and they're chauffeured off on a silver platter for your liver to break down and use as energy.

Ketones manifest in three types, all of which are somewhat hard to pronounce and spell: acetoacetate, acetone, and beta-hydroxybutyrate. The first one is important as it can be used to test your levels of ketosis, and the last two are what enters your body cells and becomes energy, beta-hydroxybutyrate being the best ketone for energy. All these molecules are taken from body fat, which can only be accessed once muscle glycogen reaches a certain depletion point. What happens is your body is essentially eating itself in the way it was designed to do, by burning through its fat reserves; it's theorized that in the past, our ancestors, hunter-gatherers, lived in a way very similar to this, as access to fresh game didn't necessarily happen every day.

The nature of how ketosis shreds the fat off your body is also interesting. For some reason yet unknown to metabolic scientists, ketosis has shown to be able to reduce the abdominal fat – fat around our viscera, our organs, better than traditional weight loss programs. This means the organs can work easier and be more free of inflammation, sparing them some of the stress that leads to type-2 diabetes, heart problems, and veritable cornucopia of other maladies. Our overall lipid profile changes as well, with a stark decline in triglycerides, reduction in LDLs, and increase in HDLs being among the most commonly observed phenomena.

One of the more "quiet" or unsung benefits of going on a ketogenic diet is the fact that the longer you stay on it, the more efficient your body gets at producing ketones and supplying you with energy from the thousands of calories stashed in your fat cells. This is the reason why many people are trying it out for the first-time crash and give up; it's not necessarily an easy or expedient thing for your body to go from a glucose-fueled system to a fat-fueled system. It takes your metabolism a while to catch up to what your mind is putting it through, but after it gets adapted, your body is rendered into a biological fat combustion engine. In addition, because your diet is composed of "heavier" foods, fats and proteins, you can feel full in what is ultimately less food and fewer calories, eliminating a need to snack and controlling your cravings. Numerous studies have proven the effectiveness of the diet, in 2012 a study conducted on obese kids and teenagers found reduced body weight, fat mass, and waist size and a reduction in shrinkage insulin levels, meaning that what they eat containing carbs won't immediately be shuttled off into their fat cells. Another study in 2017 found that a group while combining the diet with a CrossFit exercise regime, lost an average of 6 pounds of fat and improved their athletic ability over a period of six weeks.

Improved Mental Focus

Everyone and their mother's dog has gone through the stage of sleepy, heavy-headedness that accompanies consuming a whole large pizza with a side of cheesy bread and a marinara sauce with as much sugar as candy - the feared high blood sugar crash that can make it feel like you're wading through concrete. Augmented ability to cut through brain fog and focus on the task at hand is a commonly reported symptom for people in ketosis, likely explained by the fact that they're no longer in a constant, brutal cycle of eating and crashing and eating and crashing. Beta-hydroxybutyrate, one of the most important ketone bodies, might be partially responsible for this, as when it barges into your brain in all its energy-rich glory, it stimulates the growth of new mitochondria. Obviously, it can't be conclusively linked to abated feelings of fogginess, but it may explain how the diet has helped people with epilepsy, covered below.

Keto and Chronic Diseases

The original formulation for the ketogenic diet was as a way to combat epilepsy, but also has shown some success in treating maladies like diabetes, heart disease, Alzheimer's and some cancers.

The keto diet and epilepsy have shared a bed for quite some time, as that was the reason it was first brought into being. The exact mechanism of action is still poorly understood, but research at John Hopkins University shows that for children, who, for one reason or another, can't be placed on anticonvulsants, can have their seizure incidents reduced by 50% in half of the test subjects and by 90% in a third of patients. The best explanation put forth as of yet as to how it effectively sabotages epilepsy is that ketones themselves are anticonvulsant, via the fact that they are more energy efficient than glucose. The neurons in the brain adapt and increase the number of mitochondria, the powerhouse of the cell that produces energy. The increased number of mitochondria can more easily handle the massive increased energy load that flows through the brain during a seizure.

Type-2 diabetes also lays within the sights of keto's metabolic sniper rifle by draining the sugar from your blood and reducing your need for insulin and diabetes-controlling medication. To fully grasp the breadth of this, insulin resistance needs to better understood. When your cells become insulin resistant, they start refusing to take in the glucose-insulin is trying to shove into its doors, so it stays in the blood. When this happens, the pancreas goes bonkers and makes more insulin, making you a person with diabetes. A lowered insulin resistance means your body can take in the sugar like it's supposed to and your body goes back to normal.

In a study performed in 2008, over the course of 24 weeks, diabetic patients on a ketogenic diet nearly exterminated their need for medication, with 95.2% of them versus a mere 62% who were put on a low-glycemic diet. Their HDL ("Good" cholesterol) also increased, while the low-glycemic group experienced no change, and lost about 10 more pounds, losing on average 25 while the low-glycemic lost 15.

Heart disease is also treated by keto, simply because it is often linked to carrying excess weight around, which a state of ketosis helps to eliminate. In addition, inflammation from excessive carbohydrate intake, the bane of any well-functioning circulatory system, drops, freeing up huge amounts of stress on the heart and its various tendrils and valves. It should be important to note that for best heart-disease countering effects of keto; one should make sure that a higher portion of the fat they're consuming come from monounsaturated than saturated as it is rich in omega-3s, which is a great boon for the heart.

Alzheimer's Disease is a progressive form of slow dementia, usually seen in the elderly. While assuredly not a panacea for the disease that ruins lives of not only those suffering from it but from their families, certain attributes of keto can help alleviate symptoms. It has been found in animals with it that it can improve proprioception – balance, and coordination, and when supplementing with ketone esters, can reduce amyloid plaque, a characteristic marker of the disease. Again, the exact mechanism of action isn't known, and research is still ongoing. Areas of pathologic neurology are still poorly understood, probably because neurology itself is poorly understood.

Finally, some cancers, particularly brain cancers seem to respond to ketogenic diets. The theory is that the lowered blood sugar and insulin levels may reduce global inflammation, as inflammation has been known to be a root cause in many diseases. A slew of case studies found it aiding treatment of glioblastoma multiforme. Unfortunately both the most widespread and aggressive form of noggin cancer one can acquire. It is interesting to note that the diet shares a certain number of traits with fasting, most obviously autophagy, or "self-eating," the burning of fat for fuel, and both have shown some success in shrinking tumors. Perhaps it is the combination of what is basically starving out the cancer cells of easy to access energy along with the reduced global inflammation.

Oxidative stress, the accumulation of highly reactive molecules in the body without enough compounds to properly neutralize them, has been shown to lead to an increase in global inflammation. Inflammation has been linked time and time again with a slew of chronic diseases, the classical killers – diabetes, heart disease, and cancer. Antioxidants work to detoxify these free radicals; common sources are fruit and vegetables. One very interesting find was that when consuming carbohydrates alone, the body essentially switches off its natural system for handling oxidative stress, necessitating the consumption of antioxidant-rich foods. But when forsaking carbohydrates and consuming dietary fat and protein, these natural antioxidant systems are still switched on. The implications of this are immense, as it could radically change the way we look at our diets and the consumption of carbohydrates from here on out. With this in mind, it's no surprise that a diet that reduces systemic inflammation is also one that has shown some success in shutting down diseases whose root lays in inflammation.

Ketosis and Athletic Performance

Ketosis can be great for athletes of a certain type as well as people simply trying to lose weight. In particular, the ketogenic diet may be the perfect fit for endurance athletes - long-distance runners, cyclists, rowers, and swimmers. To understand why an understanding of basic exercise energy systems is important. For athletes involved in more "start and stop" type activities -- football players, wrestlers, rugby players, where one goes from 0% effort to 110% maximal effort that lasts more than 10 seconds, more easily accessible sources of energy are needed in the form of carbohydrates stored as glycogen in the muscle. Glycogen can be accessed by the body much more readily, as it's a form of energy designed for sudden powerful movements, so it's of much more use by athletes in explosive, short bouts with recovery time. High-intensity interval training, in other words. Endurance exercise is a more "steady state" form of exercise, a slow burn, so to speak. It's not particularly intense, but ideally, there are little to no breaks. The more stable nature of endurance sports lets the body chip off fat as it needs it for a slower burn activity. What may happen to a lot of runners who fuel themselves up on carbohydrates is a crash – they start out strong, running hard and fast, and then once their initial stores deplete, they're hitting a wall and lagging behind. The steady delivery of ketones to muscles keeps this problem from occurring.

Take this with a grain of salt, as a state of ketosis, when first adjusting to it, might leave some feeling sapped of energy. It's important to give yourself time to adjust before going off and trying to run the same marathon that Pheidippides ran 2500 years ago. In addition, even after achieving a state of steady ketosis where usual activities don't destroy you, to give yourself "trial runs" of a lighter exercise load than you're used to give your muscles and connective tissue time to adapt under exercise stress.

Ketosis, Food Choices, and Saving Money

One of the "soft" benefits of ketosis is thus – it lets you enjoy a rich, "regal" diet, the stuff that people usually consider the "heart" of the meal because of its wholeness and filling nature - foods like butter, meat, fish, other animal products, nuts, and whole fat dairy. Most of your calories will come from here by necessity, as they are the most fat-rich sources of nutrients unless you're interested in chugging olive oil. As a quick aside, taking shots of olive oil is not a wholly unheard-of tactic as a more extreme method of getting more healthy monounsaturated fat and filling your caloric need for the day.

When was the last time you found someone chowing down on a huge bowl of plain rice or pasta and considered it a decadent treat? And while this is a "soft" benefit, enjoying your calories from these rich and real foods without the sense of guilt that might sometimes accompany them, there is also a more "solid" benefit. It's been proven time and time again that appetites are suppressed on a low carb diet, a diet higher in protein and fat will end with you eating fewer calories. In addition, once you get used to eating a keto diet, it will be more than enough to keep your cravings for snacks away. If your diet consists of almost strictly fats, and you end up eating less of it, you'd save money on a grocery bill. In addition, you'd no longer have a desire to snack, between your body becoming more used to taking advantage of its fat stores and the fact that eating 800 calories of meat, fish, or eggs sits heavier than 800 calories of bread. In a way, this will save you time and money as well, and we all know time is money and money is time, as there's no stopping at a convenience store to pick up an expensive-per-the-calorie snack.

Wrapping It All Up

Keto's power as a diet is impressive, helping people lose weight, reduce chronic inflammation and thus fight many diseases that are ravaging our bodies, help us run, swim, row, and bike longer, and letting us enjoy a rich diet without the guilt while saving us time and money.

Chapter 3: The Bad Parts of Keto

Unfortunately, there is nothing that does not cast a shadow, metaphorical or otherwise, and ketosis has its fair share of downsides that must be considered before taking the plunge into a whole new metabolic world.

A Delicate Balance

A ketogenic diet is typically calorically broken down as 75% fat, 20% protein, and 5% carbohydrates, this is the approximate proportion – it changes depending on the person and their needs. Knowing this is all fine and dandy, but implementing it is a harder quest that requires a level of dietary dedication not seen in many people most of the time. It calls for a level of micromanagement many people are simply not willing to invest their time into, and because of this, it can be a major reason the diet fails.

Counting calories is one thing, measuring precise percentages of carbs, fats, and proteins is another. This delicate balance, if upset, will throw off the entire metabolic reaction, and, if done more incorrectly, can lead to more serious medical implications. A single miscount can throw the body out of ketosis and lead one to feel distressed and discouraged. This sort of thinking is not only hard to get into, but also hard to maintain, most medical professionals recommend that a keto diet only be maintained for a one to three months at max to take advantage of its fat-burning potential, before switching to a more "regular" diet.

Unfortunately, this can lead to Yo-yo effect, when one quickly regains the weight they lost when switching to a new diet. This is potentially more disastrous than simply being overweight, as the trauma the yo-yo effect puts on the body has been linked to increased mortality. It's not a secret that many doctors recommend that before starting a keto diet that they're consulted to test the initial health, so something needlessly tragic and avoidable doesn't happen. Oftentimes doctors recommend routine testing of ketone bodies during the diet and especially if one intends to follow it for an extended period, but that is something that can easily be done at home with the proper equipment. It's also always a good idea to talk with a nutritionist to find out the optimal macronutrient balance for you, how many calories you need in a day so you can find out how much of each nutrient you should be getting per day, and the right kinds of foods to eat while on it. Someone with a history of heart disease may want to avoid excessive saturated animal fat consumption, for instance. The overarching reality is that the ketogenic diet requires a lot of management and balancing, which many people may not be prepared to deal with.

Dietary Restrictions and Expenses

This is probably where most people falter and break, where its strength becomes its weakness. While keto does let you essentially eat, guilt-free, some of the richest foods known to man, variety is the spice of life, and if food and cooking is a major part of your life and sacrificing it isn't an option, keto simply may not be the right choice for you. It may be both a blessing and a curse that modern society has offered us such a wealth of different food that we can try at virtually any time – if we were a bunch of starving hunter-gatherers, keto would be the reality instead of merely one road that might be followed. A world without pasta, rice, bread, and candy might be too much for certain people, especially athletes who are used to fueling themselves up on such foods.

Should you be able to get over your relative scarcity of ingredients, there's the issue of "I don't know if I can whip up interesting ways to eat meat/coconut/eggs/oils/veggies 7 days a week, 3 times a day. That's a LOT of meals to come up with not a lot of ingredients, especially if you aren't interested in the culinary arts. For these people, there simply may not be enough interesting ways to eat keto and keep it up.

Cost is also to be considered. Optimally, a keto diet is one filled with healthy animal fats, foods like avocados, fresh vegetables, and olive and coconut oil. The problem with this is that for those of us who aren't dedicated to the art of savings, this can get expensive quick. It was said in the previous chapter that keto CAN save you money, the caveat here is that it CAN save you money, it potentially can, once you get used to it – if you get used to it, and still, some people simply have larger appetites than others and can eat 36 oz of steak a day and be ready for dessert afterward. If meat was once a thing you did a few times a week, having a bit of chicken breast here or there and maybe a steak or pork chops every now and then, this author finds that it can quickly burn a hole in your pocket. If you don't know how to look for deals and learn to love what's on sale, then this may be impossible for you. And if you don't have the knack to shop right and still crave variety, one might be tempted to branch into a few new hobbies, hunting, and fishing, to get your daily fat and protein needs.

The mere fact that the keto diet limits variety massively may impede many people from ever reaching ketosis in the first place, much less being able to maintain it for any significant length of time. Unfortunately, this is fundamental to the diet, as the minute you eat enough carbs to stop ketosis, you are no longer following the keto diet. While these problems with ketosis cannot be avoided, with proper supervision, there is a variety that can be, which will be covered next.

The "Keto Flu"

The transition from a carb-burning machine to a fat burning machine, especially when your body has been essentially never had the chance to do the latter before, can be a little traumatic for your biology. The keto flu is a collection of – you guessed it – flu-like symptoms that is a unique sort of misery our bodies make us suffer through as punishment for such a drastic change from what it's used to. Not everyone goes through it, but those that do feel like it's 1918 and the Spanish Flu is all the pathological rage again. It's analogous to what a heroin or nicotine addict goes through, but for carbohydrates, minus all the terrifying hallucinations and feelings of impending death (In the heroin addict's case more so than the nicotine addict's case), in other words - withdrawal.

Suffering can be mild to severe and vary by the day, making this truly "keep you on the edge of your seat" sort of misery, and can last from days to weeks. Symptoms can range to any of the following unpleasantries: nausea, vomiting, diarrhea, rapacious cravings for sugar, unexplained muscle soreness and cramping, insomnia, reduced ability to focus, stomach and abdominal cramps, dizziness, feelings of weakness, irritability, and headaches. In other words, a veritable garden of earthly delights. Thankfully, nothing lasts forever, and the keto flu is relatively harmless if one knows how to treat it.

As tempting as it may be to run a marathon or enter an impromptu cage fighting match while vomiting last night's dinner of steak with a side of coconut milk and steamed broccoli into the nearest bowl-shaped receptacle, avoiding strenuous exercise is crucial so your body can adapt to its new fuel source. Along with this is staying hydrated, as that can really help abate the feelings of cramps and help replace any fluids that may have been forced out one of your many orifices.

Along with the water, what is also lost during violent purging at one or both ends are electrolytes. Sodium, potassium, calcium, and magnesium are absolutely critical to keeping yourself on this planet as a functional human being, keeping you at a level strong enough that your boss doesn't decide to fire you for your manufactured "keto flu" disease. A loss of electrolytes can also seriously impact the kidneys in some of the most unpleasant ways imaginable, the damage can can lead to the dreaded kidney stone. Also, and less dramatically but more worrisome, overall kidney damage. Magnesium is especially essential as it assists in soothing muscle pain and ushering you off into the dreamworld. With that in mind, as in all things, getting enough sleep is also vital. Sleep is where your body makes little adjustments and modifications and repairs to assure that it is running at peak capacity, where it fixes all the damage you've done to it during the day. Without adequate sleep, doubtless one will ever fully be able to transition to a ketogenic lifestyle or even any kind of productive and healthy one.

Ketogenic Diets Can Impair Athletic Ability and Promote Muscle Wasting

For any meatheads reading this, this can be a terrifying prospect. The unfortunate reality is, as mentioned earlier, is that not every sport is designed for ketosis. Not all sports are slow burn cardio; in fact, not even most are! Many are more explosive, requiring high amounts of speed and power as well as maximal effort. Here is where ketosis lags behind – as you're barely eating any carbs, your body can't store the intramuscular glycogen it uses for fast, powerful athletic movements. What this equates to is being weaker in the field, in the weight room, or on the mats, and feeling fatigued quicker. Even if you do somehow manage to induce a shamanic trance where pain and exhaustion are mere tricks of devilish spirits, there is still the fact that adequate amounts of muscle glycogen are needed for recovery, meaning that this diet in its traditional build is not optimal for athletes. There are, of course, modifications, but this current discussion only takes into account a "traditional" ketogenic diet.

The next and more serious negative implication of ketosis is the fact that your brain cannot survive off of ketone bodies alone. The brain requires around 400 calories a day to function, around 100 grams of glucose, more if you're a genius and less if you're missing some marbles (this statement not scientifically supported). Your liver is very good at manufacturing that glucose that you need from your diet, when keto is done right, providing just enough protein and carbohydrates to be broken down into glucose to fuel your brain. The scary part happens when you miscount either of those two nutrients, undereat both of them, and eat TOO much fat, as your brain can give an executive order to your liver to start wasting away muscle tissue, which is then converted into glucose to keep itself alive. This is a relatively easy thing to avoid, as only around four ounces of protein a day are needed to avoid this, but the prospect is there.

The Possibility of Ketoacidosis

Ketoacidosis is when the count of ketones in your bloodstream reaches pathological and dangerous levels, usually only seen in a certain form of diabetes. What happens is the excessive amount of ketones turns your blood acidic, which gets deadly fast as your body exists within a very narrow pH range. The reality is that unless you really poorly mismanage your keto diet, you probably won't end up here, but it is a potential side effect that can affect your liver, brain, and kidneys. If you're following the keto diet, and someone thinks your breath smells like a strawberry that joined a street gang (In less colorful language, a "bad" sort of fruity) this can be a sign of ketoacidosis, as you exhale acetones produced by your liver. Other symptoms are pleasantries like thirst, urination, abdominal pain and vomiting, and disorientation. If you go through this, get yourself to the ER immediately because the reaper will come otherwise.

Is It Right For You?

With all of the potential failings of the keto diet now laid bare for the world and the reader to see, a necessary question must be asked: Is the ketogenic diet right for me? It can be a powerful weight management tool if used well, capable of providing scores of other health benefits that would lead to a long and happy life. But also, it's a sensitive beast, and if implemented poorly it can lead to a slew of negative symptoms. It's not for everyone, the serious athlete, the enthusiastic chef, those of us who lack the attention span and eye for detail necessary for keeping ketosis maintained and not falling off, are not necessarily good candidates, unless modifications in both the diet and lifestyle are consciously made.

Chapter 4: Getting Started with Ketosis

Now that there are no more mysteries as to what a keto diet is, its good and its bad parts, and have decided that it's right for you, you can move on to actually implement a ketogenic diet in your day-to-day life.

There's a Chinese proverb that is often abused by various motivational speakers and unengaging middle school teachers; "the journey of a thousand miles begins with a single step." Despite how tired and seemingly used up this proverb is, there is wisdom in it, as the hardest part of beginning anything new is to start doing it in the first place. Once you start something, it almost seems easier to continue. Your mental landscape shifts from "I don't even want to start it" to "I've started it, I may as well finish it," and building this kind of basic resolve is important with making a hard lifestyle change like keto, especially when it's as pervasive as it is.

Ask Yourself Why

In the first chapter, I talked about how when you're trying to get yourself off the poison of modern western diets; it's important to have a goal in mind, as it effectively serves as a road through the tangled darkness. When making a goal, one of the best ways to go about it is to approach it systematically, ask yourself questions until you know EXACTLY what you'll be doing and when, whittle your goal down like you're a man wrongly imprisoned, and the only way to pass the time is to carve chess pieces from pieces of soft rock.

In the case of this goal setting system, set yourself an overarching goal. For instance, the usual reasons for going on ketosis are "I want to lose weight," but others could include "I want to improve my endurance performance," or "I want to manage my diabetes." These are obviously vague, open goals, but that's good because there's room to grow, room to focus. This brings us to the next question in the system; "Where am I right now?" How much do you weigh right now? What is your time for a 5k right now? How many shots of insulin keeps you breathing? Once you have a reference point, you can then riddle yourself with the questions "What do I want my 5k time to be?" "How much fat do I want to lose?" "How much do I want to rely on my diabetes medication moving ahead?" Ask yourself these questions to get a more concrete handle on your goal. Once you have that figured out, you've pulled back to where you are, right now, in this current moment, you can start assessing how far you are from your goal and setting realistic steps, and take it day to day.

What changes can you make every day to reach your goal and make it a reality?

Tracking your goals

As much as we can plan and scheme, life comes at us one day at a time, so making sure that you're making these active changes in your life every day is how you're going to get where you want to go. Recording is always a good idea; if it wasn't, our scientific procedures would still be done via guesstimations and "close enough!" Recording lets you look at things from above and track your goals day to day, and from there week to week, letting you set manageable markers of progress for yourself, and then get a good idea of how long it will take you to get there. Recording must become a habit, a thing you've essentially beat into your subconscious via force of will. As an aside, there's interesting find in behavioral neurology that boils down to "Humans are most happy when they can see they are making progress on a goal, not upon reaching the goal itself."

Example plan for weight loss:

My goal is to lose weight.

How much do you weight right now?

180 pounds.

How much weight do you want to lose?

20 pounds.

How will you get there?

By following a ketogenic diet, which will put my body in a state of fat-burning ketosis, fill me heavy foods that drive down my total calorie intake and prevent me from snacking.

Okay, that sounds good. After one week of following this diet, how much have you lost? You logged it in, I hope!

2 pounds.

If you're doing this right and nothing drastic happens (losing a leg, etc.) you should be there in 10 weeks, give or take.

Another, for cardiovascular endurance:

My goal is to improve my 5k time.

What is your current 5k time?

30 minutes.

How much do you want to improve it?

By 8 minutes

How will you get there?

A ketogenic diet will help me because of the slow and steady nature of my sport, the slow burn release of energy from fat-burning ketosis fits very well as an energy system, by forsaking more carbohydrates, I avoid the carbohydrate-induced energy crash and can keep a steadier, but overall faster time.

Okay, sounds solid. After one week, how has your time improved? You've been writing it down, right?

By 1 minute.

So, reasonable, unless nothing drastic happens (again, loss of a leg may impede the ability to run somewhat) you should get there in 8 weeks, give or take.

Note: Neither of these plans is designed to be comprehensive weight loss or athletic plans, they are merely depicted here to get an idea of an efficient way to structure your goals so you can reach them.

Actually Getting Started With Ketosis

Now that that song and dance is done with, your goals are properly illuminated, and you've gotten an idea how much you'll progress per week and how keto will help you, you can move on to the meat of the problem, that being getting started with eating a ketogenic diet and living the "lifestyle."

Breaking it down:

The most important step with starting a ketogenic diet is knowing how much of each macronutrient to eat, that is the key to making a keto diet work, either way, this is going to involve some math, so pick your poison. Earlier in the book, a balance of 5% intake from carbohydrates, 20% from protein, and 75% from fat were mentioned. That means, if you're eating 2500 kcal a day, 5% will come from carbohydrates, around 125, 20% from protein, 500 calories, and the rest from fat, 1875. This obviously varies from person to person, if you're eating 3,000 or 2,000, the total amount of calories will change, but the percentage doesn't. This is where it's important to know how many calories you need per day - it depends on weight, body composition, gender, age, and activity level.

Another way to think about it, if you're more in mind of counting out servings, is grams of net carbohydrates. What are net carbohydrates, you might ask? Net profit is how much profit you've made after you've paid your loan shark off for your gambling debt and your investors for the labor on your getaway car, net carbs are a similar concept. Net carbs are the total carbs in your box of pasta or bag of spinach with the fiber subtracted from it. Why is the fiber subtracted? Because your body can't actually use fiber for calories, fiber works on you would use drain in a sink, to clean itself out. Regardless, what you want to aim for is 20 grams of net carbs or under, which can be increased the further into ketosis you get.

For the sake of clarity and consistency, the remainder of this book will use the percentage-based model.

How do I do this and what should I expect?

The keto diet isn't for everybody, and not everybody is willing to go crazy and try out scores of new foods just so they have enough variety not to go crazy and still keep themselves in ketosis. Like with anything else, it's always good to start slow and slowly ramp up the intensity. Don't go crazy and try mixing leaf lard into your coffee on your first day of keto. For one, that'll probably be gross and turn you off from it, and it's also a magnificent waste of good quality lard.

It's important to analyze and internalize a few things before going into this as well. Deep down, it's vital to know that fat is not the enemy. Fat in most of its forms is good for you and good for your heart, it's just eating the wrong kind and eating it with too much starch or sugar. Get used to cooking with more if it – pour a bit of extra olive oil or spoon some extra butter into the pan next time you fry a pork chop; it's good for you! Once you get used to it, it'll be hard to come off eating like that, trust me; it's delicious. It pays to be able to cook when doing keto as well, your ability to find a keto-appropriate frozen meal would probably be limited, expensive, and frustrating, and you can keep your taste buds and wallet happy. Do some research and try to modify some classic recipes that you're a fan of to a more keto appropriate version.

Use a classic human behavioral control system – in-group shaming, as a way to stick to your diet.

Inform your friends and cohorts of your new plan, and let them know that it's important that you experience a great dishonor from them if you sway from your diet. Social pressures are a huge motivating factor for a lot of people, use it to your dietary advantage! Finally, know what sort of disasters you're potentially in for. If you're skipping through this book and haven't read the previous chapter, there's a concise and informative (if I do say so myself) breakdown of the keto flu. Know what it is, how to avoid it if possible, and how to treat it.

Perhaps the best way to get into the keto diet isn't to one day start eating a half-dozen eggs and family's worth of bacon, but to slowly reduce carbohydrate intake over the course of a week or so. If you normally get 50% of your calories from carbohydrates, bring it down by 5% each day, compensating with increased fat, until you're down to 5%. And do this with foods you like – if you're partial to butter and fatty meat, eat some butter and fatty meat. If you're more of an avocado and eggs person, stick to avocado and eggs. Enjoy an extra couple of eggs and extra avocado instead of smearing it on toast. Before you know it, your body will be a veritable anti-fat furnace, and you'll be shedding pounds in no time, the key is to be patient and take it slow.

What to eat?

If you're like most people, your breakfast might consist of some kind of grain, maybe oatmeal or whole wheat cereal, with a side of protein and/or fruit, something to that effect. You're going to need to scrap this convention entirely if you want your body to enter starvation mode without actually starving. Certain foods absolutely need to be avoided 100% of the time from here on out, common staples like rice, corn, pasta, beans, and bread, many dairy products aside from butter, yogurt, and cheese, of course, sugar in all its nefarious forms.

What you can and should eat are things like healthy fats, olive, avocado, and coconut oils, butter, humanely-raised, and harvested lard and tallow. For protein, you should eat meat, poultry, eggs, seafood, cheese and plain, whole-fat Greek yogurt. Most or all of your carbs should come from non-starchy vegetables – no potatoes or corn. Think vegetables in the cabbage family, broccoli, cauliflower, kale, cabbage, and brussels sprouts are some of the healthiest things you can eat. Spinach, zucchini, and summer squash are also good choices; essentially, almost all vegetables are good as long as they're low in carbs.

Tying it together

Going keto can be an intimidating process, but as long as you set a comprehensive and well-structured goal plan for yourself, know what you're getting into and what to expect, as well as honing your cooking skills and what to eat, it doesn't have to be dietary torture. At the very worst, it can be an interesting experiment that may cause you to shed a few pounds – at best; it can be a complete shift in your lifestyle and perspective.

Chapter 5: Ketosis and How to Reach It

The metabolic process of ketosis is, obviously, the very core of the diet, the foundation from which all its principles stem from. What is its biological purpose? How exactly is it happening, and why is it so hard to reach? What is "optimal" ketosis, how does one get there, and how does one measure if one is in ketosis? All these questions and probably more than you thought you had will all be covered here, in this, the most technically involved and possibly dry chapter in this entire publication.

The purpose of ketosis

One of the interesting things about ketosis lies on the fact that it's such an obvious adaptation for the body, but still so hard to reach. The reality of all biological hardware is that it hates to expend energy. Expending energy is the exact opposite of what you're programmed to like doing, which is why getting up off the couch and going for a jog is so bloody difficult for a lot of people. ~~Billions of years of evolution have resulted in~~ the most complex electro-chemical structure known to science's favorite activity being loafing around and putting more energy into our systems, because who is to know when we'll need that energy to escape from a tiger or

horrible writing

rabid gang of crocodiles. Fortunately (Or unfortunately, depending on who you ask) our day-to-day is no longer subsumed by a desperate struggle for survival, so what happens when we're putting all those calories is in we get fat and unhappy.

Many dawns past, mankind had to fight just to etch out an existence in a damp cave by a river, before agriculture, and way before firearms. Food was scarce, the only thing to eat was wild game. They would feast on their flesh, and it was speculated, especially the organ meat, for its high saturation of micronutrients, and the fat, as it provided huge amounts of energy, which made it taste great. Studies done in the 19th and 20th century of the native peoples of the arctic circle show a diet that is essentially the same, and they live just fine. The dogs eat muscle meat, and the people eat fat and organs. And then, they wouldn't eat for a day or two, so their body would start to break down all the stored fat in their systems to use as energy. When hunter-gatherers settled down to become farmers, food was aplenty, but far less rich and nutrients, and this eventually became the norm. Farming would prove to be more effective for sustaining a large population, and thus the history of humanity begins there. The purpose of ketosis is to nourish the body when food is scarce, with the original signal being from a drop in blood sugar.

Mechanism of Action

Ketosis is a complex biochemical process, and the depth of it cannot be fully covered by someone who is not working in the field of biological research, but what is done here is hopefully a more demystifying explanation than previous ones found in the book that can help you fully comprehend what's going on in your body.

When blood sugar and insulin drop low from lack of carbohydrate intake, the adipose tissue, or fat cells, of the body is triggered to release stored fatty acids to be consumed as energy. This is a simple enough principle so far, but it quickly gets hairier than a gorilla who's been using rogaine. A long chain of biochemical reactions needs to take place because fatty acids can't directly enter a cell to provide with energy. They're negatively charged, so they repel away from the positively-charged cell instead of being allowed in. What happens to fix this are fatty acids need to be transformed into the compound acetyl-CoA so our bodies can utilize them as energy. There are two paths it can go down to yield energy - we're interested in one that occurs in the liver, as the mitochondria, (essentially a cell's power plant) are most efficient at transforming them into ketones than any other cell in the body. The liver cells transform acetyl-CoA by combining two acetyl-CoA molecules to form a new one, called acetoacetyl-CoA, and then with a third acetyl-CoA molecule to yield a compound called beta-hydroxy-beta-methylglutaryl-CoA, a famous spelling test word. Another enzyme then changes this mouthful of a compound to acetoacetate, one of the three different ketone bodies. Acetoacetate can then convert, via enzyme, to a second type of ketone, beta-hydroxybutyrate. Acetoacetate and beta-hydroxybutyrate are the two types of ketones that provide energy. A third type, acetone, is also produced from the degradation of acetoacetate, and is less used for energy, and is usually the ketone detected by both those who are unfortunate enough to smell keto breath and by electronic breath readers. Acetoacetate and beta-hydroxybutyrate can then be shuttled off to various parts of the body where they are broken down into their composite pieces for fuel.

How to measure your ketosis

It is possible to easily track ketosis by a variety of different means, all of which have their ups and downs. The three available on the market are blood, breath, and urine meters. Blood is the most accurate, breath can vary based on the phase of the moon, and urine's primary use is just to tell you whether you're in ketosis. From least to most effective:

Urine strips:

Again, primarily just used to tell you if you're in ketosis. There's not really an accurate count, counting pennies with your eyes closed is more reliable. However, if you're just getting into this new thing and are still gun shy about investing too much money, it's not a bad place to start, they're also far more ubiquitous than the other types. They're also fairly easy to use in compared to sticking yourself with a blood tester; you just hold the strip in the urine and the darker it is, the more ketones are in your urine, hypothetically. Problems with reliability lie in the fact that if you've hydrated yourself as doctors want, it'll show lighter as it dilutes the ketones. They're also known to be lighter in people who have been following the diet longer because the body is more efficient at hoovering up the ketones for energy.

Breath meters:

The most old school breath meter in existence is, after a week or so of ketosis, trying to give your lover a peck on the mouth. If they recoil and tell you, it smells like you've been eating fruit that went bad and started hanging out with a seedy crowd, and you've been brushing your teeth and using mouthwash, you're probably in ketosis, and what's causing that smell is acetone on your breath. However, as opposed to basing your ketone count off of how much your other half recoils, other methods take advantage of modern USB technology. You plug it in and give it a blow. The downside to this is that they can run in a very high price range, in the $200 range, and they still are not as accurate as blood meters.

Blood meter:

They say you get what you pay for, and in this case, you definitely will because while you're getting the diamond standard in terms readout of your ketosis, you'll also be paying diamond prices over a period of time if you intend on keeping the diet up for any period of time. You have to pay for each strip, and they run about a buck a strip, which adds up fast. There is the chance of failed readings, but as long as you're accurate with your pricking you should be fine, but it does mean you might waste a dollar here and there. Downsides are obvious besides long-term price, and not everyone has what it takes to prick themselves in the finger.

Interpreting readings:

When you get a reading of ketone count, it'll be somewhere between 0 and 3 mmol/L.

- .5 and below doesn't count as ketosis; your body is running as normal

- .6 to 1.5 you're there, but it's light.
- 1.5 – 3.0 is your best ketosis, where you want to be to burn through the most weight.
- 3 and onward is not really necessary; it more often can indicate prolonged fasting/starvation periods than anything else. You aren't going through any more calories than those in the 1.5-3.0 range. However...
- 6 – Anything approaching this means you're getting into ketoacidosis, which can be potentially fatal. It's rare that you would reach that, but in case you do, seek medical attention immediately.

Attaining optimal ketosis

Ketosis is not a quick metabolic state to get into, as it takes your body burning through all its saved-up glucose and then it starts to break down your fatty acids. This can take up to 2 to 3 days of fasting or conscious eating on a ketogenic diet to get to. And when it begins, it's not exactly the most efficient process. It can take up to two weeks for your body to start utilizing beta-hydroxybutyrate in amounts considered strong enough to fend off the feeling of impending death from the keto flu, which is why when you enter ketosis, it's crucial to stick with it for a few days to assure that your body can adapt and take full advantage of its capability to produce energy for you.

Reaching optimal ketosis is essentially the same thing as reaching lite ketosis. It's just a manner of patience and delicate balance of nutrients.

You still need glucose and how your brain is fueled

Many parts of the body can't live off ketone bodies alone; they still require a fair bit of glucose to keep functioning, your brain most importantly. Fats are composed of fatty acids and glycerol, and while the fatty acids can be used to form ketones, the glycerol is metabolized by your liver through gluconeogenesis to form new glucose for your brain. Hearty contributions from lactate and amino acids are also to thank for producing glucose. Normally, as you undergo ketosis, your brain starts off only getting around 30% of its energy from the ketones, but as ketones meet and greet and become chummy with parts of your anatomy, that will rise to 70%, and it prefers beta-hydroxybutyrate, which, if you recall, is also the compound that helps the neurons develop more mitochondria, to deal with its increased energetic load.

Regardless, about a third of your brain will still sequester itself off and refuse to mingle with its new sources of energy, and that's where gluconeogenesis comes in. Your brain is the most selfish organ in your body and thinks of itself more highly the "lower" organs, so all the glucose you're producing from the glycerol and proteins and your small amounts of carbs are going right there. That's how your brain stays fed on keto, by stealing from the rest of your body. But remember, the wrong amount of protein and not enough fat can throw it off. This is sort of where it gets tricky. You need to get enough protein in to prevent your muscles from wasting and maintain your brain health, but not too much to throw you out of it. That's why it's so incredibly important to make sure that you're getting exactly what you need and staying stuffed with fat instead of more meat/eggs/fish.

Conclusion:

Ketosis is a complex biochemical process that comes about from a cascade of reactions with a lot of long, garbled names, and a lot of enzymes that weren't named here, but ends up in a magnificent process that can be abused for weight loss purposes. Doubtless, our hunter-gatherer ancestors never could have conceived of such a world, where food was so abundant that we had to manipulate our bodies into starving ourselves without the starvation aspect, nor a world where it was so easy to track and measure your starvation for optimal weight loss, but the future is truly a magnificent place, and with modern technology, reaching optimal ketosis for optimum weight loss is as easy as a prick of the finger.

Chapter 6: Making Keto Work for Everybody

This chapter should begin by admitting that "everybody" is a misnomer; you can't make anything work for everybody, there's always some miniscule percentage that has reasons as to why they can't. Sometimes, their simple inherent biology isn't compatible with it, or they can't stand the dietary restrictions, or because of a sport they play or their job, they need the quicker energy supplied by carbohydrates. But keto can still work for virtually everybody, provided they have the discipline and the know-how.

Keto on a budget

Reaching ketosis is a double-edged sword. Unless you're starving yourself, your diet is massively different than what you're used to, and let's be realistic here, a diet heavy in fat, high-quality oil, meat, and vegetables can add up quickly. There's a reason that we sometimes refer to the carbs and fibrous roughage on our plates as the "filler food," because it's cheap and abundant and fills you up. Whether you're a poor college kid, in between jobs or trapped at a bad gig or just a penny-pincher, it's easy to eat keto on a budget as long as you keep your head in it.

The first thing to remember is that if you're eating more fat, you're going to be less hungry inherently, so you don't have to refuel between meals or snack constantly, and hey, you might even be able to skip a meal or two. Less snacking and less time eating by itself is a money-saving strategy. You will also find that a large reason as to why we feel hungry is purely from adaptation – your stomach is accustomed to being fed whenever it wants, so it gets spoiled, when really, missing a meal won't render you an emaciated skeleton, not when you have plenty of energy stored away.

And just because you're on keto doesn't mean that you have to start buying grass-fed steak in massive qualities, just as long as you're getting enough protein, breaking the bank isn't necessary.

Tips for keeping your wallet and belly full

- First off, as a universal rule when it comes to buying groceries, consider buying in bulk. Buying in bulk is usually cheaper per pound or per ounce provided you know how to preserve your goods; it will save you many a trip to the grocery store. This especially applies to things like coconut and olive oil, you can buy a huge jug, and as long as it's capped right, it will last for months.

- Consider shopping at farmer's markets, usually the smaller, the better. Anything that has grown to resemble a state fair with a lot of cooked food vendors generally has higher prices. People are more open to bargaining, and certain in-season vegetables can come much cheaper. If you catch a deal, even meats and other animal products can be cheaper than the bigger stores, and usually better raised as well.

- Immigrant stores are similar; most of them have certain keto-friendly foods, eggs, chicken, oils, and the like marked down compared to the more "vanilla" stores.

- When looking for animal proteins, skip the steak and go for the tougher, cheaper cuts. Whole picnic hams, pork shoulder roasts, whole beef chuck roast and brisket, and whole chickens are cheaper than their broken-down forms. Chickens are easy to break down once you get the swing of it and can be cooked in bulk and frozen. Anything off the skeleton that you don't eat can be saved and boiled in a pot to make stock to use for later.

- If in-season low-carb produce is still expensive, buy it frozen. Frozen produce is still just as nutrient dense as regular produce and comes in huge bags. Avoid canned, as they're usually so hard-boiled than they manage to sap the nutrients out of them.

- If you can get past it, consider eating organ meats. This also might be a good thing to look out for at a farmer's markets. Ask your local farmer what he does with his offal, and if it's within your budget and you're feeling adventurous give it a try. Offal is oftentimes more nutritious in a lot of ways than "regular" meat, so in addition to meeting your keto goals, you'll be getting a lot of micronutrients as well.

- When it comes to offal, it helps to dip your toes in the water before going all out and buying a whole pig head or something similarly ghastly. Try making stock with pig feet, as they're filled with healthy collagen. If you can get past that, try out tongue and heart. They're essentially the same kind of muscle you're used to eating, just in a more familiar shape. Tongue is fantastic braised and heart is great seared in a pan and sliced thin. The liver has a stronger taste, but soaked in milk and cooked right can be evened out. If it's still too much, mix it in with some ground meat – pork is almost always cheaper, and ground heart is cheaper than that.

- Get familiar with cheese and eggs. Cheese is a fantastic source of protein and fat, and a little goes a long way, and eggs are cheap and very nutritious. Certain cheeses can even be cooked in a pan to form a kind of keto flatbread or cracker, with the same crunch but made from cheese.

- Finally, if you can't cook, learn how to. Know your seasonings; they're a good investment to help null the pain of repetitive meals. Find out what you like and what goes on what – for instance, what I've learned as an enthusiastic home cook is that garlic apparently goes good on everything. Eating out is expensive, even at cheap places, and oftentimes they won't be able to account for your diet. If you can throw together a good keto meal from chicken livers, a can of tomatoes, garlic, and a half cup of coconut oil, you're probably about three steps ahead of most people.

Keto and the holidays

I know it's the holidays because I can feel every cell in my gastrointestinal system screaming for mercy from the nuclear carbohydrate bomb I've forced dropped on it. Something about the holidays really gets people eating like crap – the cold weather, the abundance of food, the sense of comfort and security from being around your family. These factors all combine into a nightmarish wraith that will chase you down (mentally) stuffing cookies and pasta and panettone down your throat and won't rest until a couple of notches has loosened your belt loop. Fear not – for there are ways to banish this wraith back to the sugary hell from whence he came.

The first and foremost thing to remember is self-control. Unless you are running the entire holiday show and making ALL THE FOOD, you can't control what your friends and family will bring, but you can control what you actually put in your piehole. Grandma will probably not change her 400-year-old Bavarian pastry recipe because the grandkid whose name she can't remember is following some strange new diet. Keep in mind why you're following this diet, keep your goals in mind, and what step you're on to reach them. You are in charge of you. Only you can make you eat that cookie or hunk of bread. It's a thousand times easier not to eat something than to endeavor to burn it off later.

Center your activities around things besides eating. As a culture, I think it's collectively fine to admit that the food is half the reason we are all still at peace during the holidays. It keeps us happy and sedated and makes our great aunt's rambles about the depression a little easier to sit through. But there are other activities – talk to your family, help them cook so you can sneak in your own creations. Play a ball game, go caroling, pumpkin carving, pumpkin throwing, volunteer in a soup kitchen, something that doesn't revolve around food.

When it comes to the table though, bring something that is in the clear for your gut. Roasted green vegetables or a salad, bring a meat dish, something that you know you can come back to if the turkey is double-breaded and the only side is candied yams. Realistically, they won't be like that and take advantage of the wealth of food around you. Good chance that somewhere around the dinner table there's something that fits your diet pick and choose the meat and green vegetables.

It's also important to know where carbs could be lurking in ambush - gravy is basically an emulsion of the best things in life – fat, flour, and meat broth, but the flour kicks you out of your diet. If the turkey is drier than the desert, opt for the dark meat, always richer in taste, micronutrients, and fat. You can even try making a ketogenic version of a holiday classic if you feel like flexing your ability and showing off your flashy new diet to your old relatives who still communicate via telegram.

Finally, if your resolve breaks and you start reaching for the rolls and rice, stick to those closest to your heart, (Your gut?) so you can truly appreciate it. Set a limit ahead of time, but while you're eating it, savor it, because both of us know this is the last you'll get for a while.

Keto and going out

Everyone likes a night on the town, but how do you properly impress your date with your nutritional awareness and stick to your diet? Is it possible to stick to keto and still embarrass yourself on the dance floor after a bit too much alcohol? This section aims to answer these questions.

What do I order?

Obviously, avoid the complimentary bread, skip out on the pasta, and don't eat dessert. But there is more finesse to it – many restaurants will let you replace your starch with a side vegetable or salad instead, so keep your eyes open for that option. If you're a hip enough burger joint, you can get it wrapped in lettuce like a little burgerrito hybrid. If you can't avoid the starch with your meal, try forcing it on your friend, or simply not eating it and tossing it in the trash, so the temptation isn't there.

Many places, sandwich joints in particular, usually offer a salad with a protein instead of a bread. Opt for that instead, and add extra fat where you can. Ask for a splash of olive oil on your steamed veggies, or an extra serving of dressing for your salad. Remember to ask the waiter about the nutritional content of anything not properly explained, finding extra sugars in salad dressings is very common. If they don't have a proper healthy dressing, simply ask for olive oil and vinegar. Always drink water or unsweet tea or coffee with your meals.

Alcohol

Alcohol is a whole different ball game. Beer and wine both are filled with carbs, so those are right out, and if you're partial to living in the moment with sugary cocktails despite the hangover they give, I have bad news for you. You'll have to resort to only drinking hard liquor and water to get the courage to ask the girl/guy on the sidelines out, anything else doesn't fit. Certain cocktails might fit, drinks with pickle or olive brine are in the clear, but generally, if it tastes good, spit it out. There is an upside, as a night of all spirits and water is possibly the "cleanest" most efficient and cost-effective way to get drunk, even if it's not pleasant. On the downside, it's all too real a fact that alcohol lowers inhibitions, so be careful not to have too much and drink responsibly.

Keto while traveling

It's perfectly possible to maintain your diet while globetrotting, but knowing the background of where you're going is vital. Some countries and locations follow a diet with a higher carbohydrate count than others, and it's important to get informed and find out alternatives before you go. The same principles apply as when going out, just on a larger scale. If your vacation is more active, hiking the Appalachian trail, you're going to need energy. Make sure to keep this in mind when packing your trail food. The perfect food for this sort of activity would be pemmican, a native American trail food made of dried meat and fat. If you can't find it or make it, many stores sell salami and other cured meats. Cured and smoked meats are not the best foods for you, but the kinds that preserved more traditionally tend to have less of a damaging effect, and it keeps you in ketosis and not starving, which is the most important thing.

It can work for (virtually) everybody

Keto is a powerful weight loss tool that, with some knowledge and discipline, can work for those of us on a budget, going out, traveling, and during the holidays. It's not easy – but doing something worth it rarely is, but it's easily possible once you apply what you learned in this chapter.

Chapter 7: Is Keto a Good Fit for You?

In the last chapter, we talked about how ketosis can potentially work for everybody, but that doesn't necessarily mean it's the best diet for *everybody*. This chapter encourages you to reflect on your lifestyle, in all its facets, to see if this new trendy diet will fit you. All the pieces that define who you are - your current diet, occupation, your ethnic and religious background, where and who you live with, personality, social relations, and activity level provide you with the answer to the question "is this is the right diet for me?"

One thing to keep in mind is that if you're interested in the diet and are confident you can reach ketosis, try it out. See how you feel, see if you think it can be a viable option, provided everything else in your life is in alignment. You won't know until you try, you might get on the diet and lose the weight you've been trying to lose for the last year and feel great and energized. If by some chance, you fall off the wagon and the issue wasn't you're your willpower, no harm done, you tried it, and factors outside your control means it didn't work for you. That's how things happen sometimes.

Personality

This is the most important factor of all, knowing yourself and your behaviors. If you know, you're the kind of person who can't resist a cookie or just loves pasta to an unhealthy degree, start rethinking your dieting options. Even lacking a detail-oriented personality can put you in a bind, as it's a very sensitive diet. Let's re-establish this now - keto is not for all types of people, simply because it requires a lot more conscious decision making and planning than what we're used to when it comes to food. Not everyone is like that, and that's okay. Calculating a percentage of fat, protein, and calories to eat everyday and then revamping your eating habits around them isn't exactly rocket science, but it's still a hassle for most of us. If you have problems resisting temptation, or if food is a comfort and a passion for you, or the way you pay your bills, these can all conflict. And it helps to be experienced in dieting – if you've counted calories before, if you've gone on a prolonged fast, or if simply nothing else has worked for you, and you're getting desperate, you might excel on this diet.

Regimented people who are more interested in form and results than taste probably will end up doing better on this diet as well. Openness is one of the "big five" personality traits, and more open people are always interested in trying new things. If you're a very open person who likes variety, what boils down to cutting yourself off from an entire food group and pigeonholing you into a small window would quickly drive you up a wall from monotony and cause you to break your diet.

Current diet

How you eat right now is important, which is why, if you're interested in ketosis, it's important to ask yourself why you want to go on it. If your current diet works for you and you're living with no problems, weight or otherwise, why try to change it? Curiosity is certainly a factor, and by all means, try it if you want, but don't try to force it if it doesn't work like you thought. If you need to have your meals with a glass of oil instead of water, there's a red flag.

If you're interested in the diet but don't need all health benefits it can yield, it could be a better idea to try out a "lite" version of it, the low-carb diet, or try fasting. The low-carb diet will yield the same sensation of fullness as keto that leads to fewer calories consumed. Fasting is an excellent technique for weight management, changing your relationship with food, building self-control, has the benefit of spiking growth hormone, known for its anti-aging properties. But, at the end of the day, if your current diet is chock full of carbs and you're living just fine, it might not be worth it to go into ketosis.

Activity level and type

If you're a football player, fighter, rugby player, or any athlete whose sport is based on anaerobic systems of producing energy, you should rethink your decision. You're going to need a lot of carbohydrates going into those muscles to keep everything functioning as best it possibly can. If you're working out hard in high-intensity intervals several days a week, being on ketosis can make you feel like you're circling the drain. But if you're a runner who's putting in 6 miles a day, this could be the perfect fit. Even people who walk a lot, for work or pleasure, can make good use of ketosis. Weight training lies somewhere in between a properly adapted weightlifter might feel fine on ketosis or even fasted and be able to pull like they always do. The issue is if you were interested in starting off weightlifting and tried doing it during keto, the proper physiological adaptations would not have occurred, and you wouldn't be able to perform anywhere near your best.

Where you live and who you live with

Eating keto, even if you're doing it on a budget, can get expensive, especially if you want to indulge in something besides organ meat and drinking a cup of oil every now and then. Certain parts of the country – and certain parts of the world, of course, may have extremely inflated food prices or simply poor access to ketogenic foods. If you're living in a more rural area of an underdeveloped country, most of the options for food are probably starchy, as they're the easiest to grow in mass. It may be possible to eat a ketogenic diet, but it may not be worth the trouble and extra time investment, or you may not be able to get your macronutrient balance right every day. Other places may be "food deserts" where access to fresh and unprocessed is very limited or impossible. While eating keto may be possible on a diet of slim jims and hotdogs, it's not healthy or affordable.

If you have housemates who drink often or eat your food (hopefully, buddies of yours), maybe you live a bit more "communally" than the average home, that would also be a problem. Peer pressure is a very real and very effective phenomenon. Having social pressures every single day can quickly wear down even the most resolved dieter. Or they may sometimes eat your food, but in return, offer you a slice of their pizza - something to that effect - and you figure some food is better than no food, right? In addition, snacks or alcohol laying around everywhere can be a temptation that you don't need. On the flip side, living with your parents can also make it a challenge unless you're willing to take matters of cooking into your own hands. Coming home to a comforting home-cooked meal every day is an alluring pull, not even counting on the advanced form of social pressures parents can use.

Type of employment

Different types of jobs have different caloric needs and stress levels, and stress affects eating. Not to disparage any career choices, but jobs like doctor, nurse, heavy equipment operator are generally more stressful than a receptionist or a writer. A lot of people stress eat, and a lot of people are stressed out because of their job, and stress eating often leads to poorly thought out choices. Amount of physical exertion at work is a factor as well. Consider the manual laborer, he or she might be performing the same kind and level of activity as an athlete, the kind of person who moves bricks all day or swings a sledgehammer will need an energy source that can provide for these big, powerful movements. Meanwhile, someone who sits a chair for four to five hours at a time will need fewer calories and can probably perform fine just breaking down their own fat. In fact, the ketogenic diet would probably greatly aid someone like that as sitting has been linked to high mortality, probably via the accumulation of excess weight.

Ethnic/cultural background

Some of the most powerful cables in the world that bind us come from our families. They're the cradle of our personality. They fostered us, it gives us a context as to where we came from so we can know where we're going and get the impression that we're a part of something bigger than ourselves. In a more practical sense, the foods we eat are massively affected by how we grew up and what we can cook competently, or at least, make not taste like death. Even if you don't live with or around your family anymore, the imprints they made are as fissures in you, massive and unavoidable. Someone from India would be more predisposed to following a vegan or vegetarian diet, chocked full of naan bread and lentils. An Italian would have been eating pasta and pizza since he was a boy. Sometimes it's just hard to make the jump into a new diet where you're not confident that you'll be able to feed yourself without wanting to vomit up three times the amount of oil you're used to consuming at once.

Religion is also a factor for a lot of people. As the genesis of society itself lies in grain farming since time immemorial bread has been intrinsic to religious rituals. This is observed in almost every mass organized religion worldwide. Imagine how awkward it would be to tell your priest that you can't take communion because you're doing keto? Many religions have strict rules about what you can eat and when, and if you're a true devout this can be problematic as you must choose between spirituality and diet. If there can be no compromise brokered, that would be a problem moving ahead. The only alternative would be to create your own religion centered around the keto diet, which probably would have some kind of root in primitive mysticism and animism that would necessitate shamanic trances, which is a whole different can of worms.

Social life

The final thing to be considered is your gang of miscreants you chum around with. Would they be supportive, or would they chide you about your new diet and actively discourage you? Would they take it a step further, and actively dump sugar onto what you're eating without telling you, and sneak breadcrumbs into food they said with keto? For starters, if you have friends like that, they probably are not very good friends, and you should consider getting new ones. But if your friends are actually normal and the worst they do is tease you about it, it could be worth it to have a talk with them and let them know that you're trying to improve yourself, and if they're worth their salt, they'll understand and desist. However, if you are all a bunch of raving party animals and going out on the town is a common occurrence, this could also lead to trouble. As alluded to earlier, drinking will lower inhibitions. In addition to just being plain not very good for you overall, if you have many bouts of drinking over the course of a month, there's a realistic chance that might break your diet at some point. Think about your habits, your friend's habits, because they will affect you, and consider whether keeping your relationship as it is might sabotage your diet. The best solution would be adaptation on their end and your end, with both working to making you happy, but obviously, this can't always happen.

So, is it realistic for you?

Once you consider these factors, everything from family to personality, social life to activity, you'll be properly equipped to know if this is the move for you. There's no perfect diet for everyone, and everyone is different. If you decide to try out the keto diet and find that it's not for you, there's no harm in going back to the drawing board and trying out something new to see if it will get the results you're looking for, just don't be too hard on yourself and try to sustain something unsustainable. Remember to really ruminate on these factors, because while you may be a lapsed Catholic jogger who works in an office, and that really seems like a good fit for someone going on a diet, if you're used to shotgunning beers with your boys on the weekends, your liver will be too occupied cleaning you out to make ketones.

Chapter 8: Exercise and Keto

Ketosis and exercise may initially seem like a poor combination. Exercise, by necessity, requires a lot of carbohydrates for energy, right? Well, not exactly. Scores of professional athletes have had great results on ketosis, and it's true that they're genetically blessed, have a ridiculous work ethic, and the best coaches, dieticians, and doctors money can buy, but with the right head on your shoulders, there's no reason why you can't excel on the field or in the weight room while keeping the fat-burning engine lit. There's a real downside that's been alluded to previously, and it's that unfortunately, ketosis and high-intensity training don't mix, because no matter what you do, it's powered by glycogen, which is made from carbohydrates, or at least not traditional ketosis, with a modified plan, results can be had. There are still plenty of other modalities to follow, though. Supplementation should also be rethought, as the change in your macronutrient profile will doubtless change what you need and what you don't need.

A few considerations

To really understand what this chapter is going to dive in to, a basic understanding of your body's energy systems is needed. To keep it short and sweet (or short and fatty, I guess) your body has three main energy systems for exercise. Ketosis really does good for one of them.

From shortest to longest duration of activity, there is the phosphagen system, the anaerobic system, and the aerobic system. The phosphagen system is used for heavy weightlifting - it's for very short, powerful movements. This isn't affected by ketosis because it's neither glucose fed nor fat fed, it's something else entirely. A good way to remember how the phosphagen system works is by thinking of it as any very powerful movements that last under 10-12 seconds. In other words, it's irrelevant and if you happen to be a world class powerlifter/golfer you can go on keto and survive the workout.

The anaerobic system is used for 10 seconds to up to a minute or more, depending on the athlete, of all-out maximum effort activity like wrestling, boxing, team sports, the more "sporty" sorts of sports. This system gets hit the hardest by ketosis, and while you probably can go keto and do some of this, you're going to feel like Jacob wrestling God in the desert after. This is potentially doable, but there's a good chance of reduced performance, and you may have to tweak your diet a fair bit to get it to work, this will be covered later on.

The final system is aerobic, which after a few minutes starts knocking on the door to your fat cells to ask for donations to its starving muscle tissue. It burns through the stored up glucose in your muscles, but nowhere near to the degree that anaerobic activity does. This system is least affected by ketosis it's functioning fairly similarly to how your body works naturally anyway.

Remember that going into ketosis takes time, and at first, you may feel less like a sleek fat-eating machine and more like a person covered in grease who can't think straight. This will resolve - eventually, your body will adapt, and you will find a way to wash the butter from your last meal off your hands. It's good to wait until you feel back to your old self again before trying to do your run or pull your usual deadlift, which shouldn't be too hard as my motivation to crush weight and cross-country run is dampened when I feel like my brain has been transformed into concrete.

Once you feel like you can walk across the room without getting lost, don't go nuts, keep your workouts familiar. Physiological adaptations happen over time to the body to be good at a certain physical skill; tendons strengthen, muscle cross-sectional area increases, the heart, and lungs get more powerful, your body knows what it's doing. But if you try to get into ballistic cross country skiing instead of your usual round in the weight room, things may not end up so pretty. In addition, if you change too much at once, regardless if you succeed or fail, there are too many variables at play to tell you why and how it worked or didn't work.

Make sure your calories are where they need to be. Keto is notorious (or famous, more positively) for keeping appetite down, which is great if you're going to be watching TV all day or playing solitaire while pretending to be working, but not so great if you're trying to swim the English Channel. If you're going to be exercising you really need those calories and all your fat. So chow down on that last bag of pork rinds before the race, you'll need it.

How to change your body composition

For a lot of people, shedding fat is the primary objective of exercise. Well, that's great news, because the ketogenic diet is designed for that, and double powerful when combined with exercise. As you know, when performing bouts of aerobic exercise, glycogen is partially bypassed in favor of delicious fatty ketones, meaning that when you exercise in ketosis, you're really speeding up that autophagy of fatty tissue during and after exercise.

Weightlifters, bodybuilders, and any number of other athletes often have to change weight classes for a meet or show. For putting on weight, aim to eat an additional 300 calories a day from fat. The inverse is the same – for losing weight, drop 300 to 500 calories a day, from both dieting and exercise.

It is still *extremely* important to eat enough protein as if you don't, your body will go delusional from lack of carbohydrates and start seeing your muscle as a sugary treat, almost identically to how cartoon characters would see each other as ice-cream sundaes when trapped on a desert island. A good metric to go by for those athletes looking to pack on muscle is **one gram per pound of bodyweigh**t, enough to keep your muscle from wasting away and keep you growing. Usually, I recommend figuring out your protein requirements first and basing the rest of your daily nutrition around that. However many grams protein you eat will be that 20% or of your daily intake, and thus fat and carbohydrates are adjusted for it.

To give you a live demonstration of how to eat to try to pack on muscle; on a 2,000 calorie diet, if you're eating 100 grams of protein a day, which is 400 calories, and 20% of your daily calories, you'd need to eat an additional 166 grams of fat, about 1500 calories. The last 100 calories should come from carbs to fill in the last 5%, 25 grams.

Note that this is most likely not enough for the average bodybuilder to put on weight, but is merely meant to show you how to properly structure your diet when you're trying to pack on muscle.

Modifying your plan

If doing both keto and continuing to wrestle is unavoidable, consider how you're going to eat. One modification of the ketogenic diet is called the targeted ketogenic diet and it - now don't spit out your steak - briefly throws you out of ketosis for the purposes of exercise performance. Your muscles need that quick-acting fuel to be able to contract right, right? Right! But if you time it, so you're eating anywhere from 25 to 50 grams of carbs, a light to moderate amount, before you work out, along with some protein, anywhere from an hour to half an hour beforehand, it should give you the boost you need to not feel like an Egyptian slave building the pyramids. It's actually beneficial if you want to keep your muscle quality as high as possible if you're doing this as well because your old buddy insulin comes out of his den to move glucose into the cells, and he also has the added benefit of slowing muscle degradation during your workout.

For the really dedicated amongst us, it helps even to know what kind of sugar to eat. Dextrose and glucose are the ones that are taken in an express train right to your muscles, usually found in candy than in fruit, so it's an excuse to eat that piece of candy you found under your car seat a week ago. If you want to be really precise, glucose gel packets are also available, or some kind of sugary sports drink works as well because they also contain electrolytes which you're going to be going through at a fast during exercise.

Finally, it's a good idea always to have a good amount of protein after a workout, as that is when your body's sensitivity to it is highest, and you need it the most to fuel your muscular restructuring and prevent any breakdown of existing muscle tissue.

You may be wondering if knocking yourself out of ketosis will mean you have a hard time getting back in. The short answer is no, as long as you follow the diet after your workout you'll be getting your ketone count back up in no time, provided you didn't eat too many carbs in the first place. The longer answer is still no, but there are things you can do to mitigate your brief visit with the old you. Steady-state mild cardio, maybe a fast walk or slow jog, has been shown to lower insulin levels. Have a refreshing chug of MCT, medium-chain triglyceride oil, sometime before, during, or after your workout, as MCTs are repurposed into ketones in no time. The reality of all this is that it is largely irrelevant, as long as you follow the diet you'll go back into ketosis just fine, and there are a bunch of different factors to see if you even left it in the first place. How hard and long you worked out will change it, probably putting you back in if you burned through your carby treat, and how long you've been in ketosis in the first place matter a lot.

Ketosis and weightlifting

For the average joes, it's important to know which training style yours mostly resembles and work from there. A ketogenic diet can work in harmony with weightlifting, but it depends on what kind of weightlifting you're doing and the twisting of a few factors.

Different schools of movement

As easy as it would be to say "ketosis and weight lifting" are compatible or not compatible, it is unfortunately not so cut and dry. For starters "weightlifting" is something of deceiving term, as it can vary depending on the athlete. In a strict sense, "weightlifting" refers to Olympic weightlifting, a sport centered around two major lifts and accessory movements to those lifts. Olympic weightlifting's two lifts are the clean and jerk and the snatch. Olympic weightlifting is a high-skill sport, with both lifts requiring exceptional balance and mobility, not to mention loads of explosive power. In general, it uses the phosphagen system the most.

Another common type of training is powerlifting, which is centered around three lifts, the bench press, squat, and deadlift. Powerlifting is less technically demanding and less explosive (Powerlifting still requires tons of explosive strength, but the movements are by nature never as dynamic or quick as Olympic movements.) but rewards brutal, slow strength, and also makes great use of the phosphagen system, doubtless with bleed in from the glycogen-fed anaerobic system.

Bodybuilding also falls under the umbrella of "weightlifting," and Arnold Schwarzenegger doing bicep curls in a state of ecstasy is probably what most non-athletes picture when the word "weightlifting" is said. Unlike powerlifting and Olympic lifting, bodybuilding is not about how high your total with two or three exercises is. Bodybuilding is about trying to get your muscles as big as possible, which bodybuilding is a far more open training style than Olympic lifting or powerlifting. Training is more focused on set ranges of repetition and rest times that are designed to maximize muscular hypertrophy - the size of the muscle. To achieve this, bodybuilding needs to maximize time under tension. To water down years of scientific research to an easy-to-remember maxim, the more time under tension - the time your bicep is contracted while curling a weight - the bigger they get. Bodybuilders manipulate their physiology by using moderate weight with higher-repetition sets and a short rest time to maximize their muscle growth by maximizing how long they're contracted for. This range can be where from 8 to 12 reps, with rest times lasting anywhere from 30 seconds to two minutes and weight anywhere from 50% to 75%. There may be some commonalities amongst bodybuilder programming, but they tend to vary person to person more so than powerlifting or Olympic lifting would. Because of the nature of having to get every muscle in the body as large and symmetrical as possible, bodybuilding training times might run longer than powerlifting or Olympic lifting. Bodybuilding will use the phosphagen system for its heavier lifting, and for its burnout muscle-stressing movements, will make more use of the anaerobic system.

With all this in mind, for the average dieter and weight enthusiast, it's doubtful that they strictly train like any of these athletes, which is where things get hairier. Each of these training styles stresses a different energy system more than the other, with bodybuilding probably doing the best job at depleting muscle glycogen and Olympic lifting relying the most on the phosphagen system and powerlifting hanging out in the middle. It's important to know how you're going to train. Doing high repetition exercises would fall under the glucose-fed system, things like 8-12 reps, and when your muscle glycogen is low, your results will suffer.

How do I apply this?

Now that we have an idea of what kinds of lifting are out there, we can think about our goal. If you're looking to develop a lot of power and strength, usually with rep ranges in the 1 to 5 range, the domain of Olympic lifting and powerlifting, and you've already adapted to your new diet, you can safely assume that you'll be able to keep working out unhindered.

If your style is more bodybuilding or mixed style, with a lot of variations in things like exercises from day to day and rep ranges and rest times and a longer workout, you might feel like you're being put through a strange form of self-induced torture. Your body is going to need extra glycogen, because every time you do a set of high-rep bicep curls or lunges, your body starts tapping into its glycogen-fed system, which you have depleted because of your diet. If you want to excel and your workout has a bunch of these high-rep movements, consider eating your carbs before you work out to give yourself the energy to keep yourself from passing out on a strenuous lift.

It should be noted that all training types use all energy systems to some degree. It could be said, for example, that 80% of Olympic-style training uses creatine phosphate for fuel, but physiology is never that cut, and dry and inevitably other systems will be used to smaller degrees. For example – many programs based around developing power usually have a fair amount of "bodybuilding-style" accessory work to assure that all the helping muscles in the lift are also up to top shape, and oftentimes these rep ranges can exceed the usual for 1 to 5 reps power and thus expire the creatine phosphate-fed system and start tapping into the glycogen system. If this has been happening to you, remember your body talks to you, and if you're suffering through your power-focused workout, you should consider following the targeted ketogenic diet and supplement with carbs 30 minutes to an hour before your workouts.

Ketosis and cardio

Ketosis and cardio really are a fantastic couple and have been bedmates maybe even going back to before recorded history. As a quick aside, consider what might have been the human condition throughout history, and even exists today in parts of the world. We are weaker and smaller than many animals, but some reason we still derive a lot of nutrients from their flesh. We are smart and well-adapted for endurance running, though our pace is slow, we could usually run megafauna to exhaustion. Our bodies can take that stored fat and toss it right in our furnace to keep our legs pumping so that one day, we might wipe the mammoth scourge off the face of the planet. Nothing has changed nowadays, we're still great at it, but we're much lazier and would rather just shoot it.

Activities that count as cardio would be triathlete's events, jogging, cycling, swimming, rowing, the elliptical, and dance classes. Nothing that winds you and makes you want to throw up, essentially.

If you primarily exercise by doing steady-state, unchanging submaximal cardio, defined as getting you to within 50-70% of your maximum heart rate, ketosis fits in a whole lot easier with many less dietary shenanigans than weightlifting. What's my maximum heart rate, you may ask? The shorthand for it is generally 220 minus your age. Once again, nothing is set in stone as everyone's physiology is different, but that's a good ballpark marker to go for. So if you're 27, it would be anywhere from 97 to 135 beats per minute.

If you're already a cardio athlete, once you've adapted, you're good to go. But still, take things slow. Lower your intensity than what you're used to and work your way back up. Intensity, for cardio, is defined as your heart rate. If you're a carbohydrate-fed cardio athlete, who has gamed their heart rate to be able to operate at 70%, drop it down to 60% or 50% and try to make it your usual time. If you feel good, great; you've successfully managed to make the jump. If not, don't get discouraged. Wait a few more days and try it again, your body might need more time to flood fatty acids into your bloodstream.

If you're new to cardio and keto, and which case, you're probably looking to lose a lot of weight, congratulations on taking the first steps, and when you inevitably feel like there's an invisible metabolic vampire sapping you of energy after your first keto-fed session on a treadmill, the pain does abate. It takes a few weeks for a regularly-fed person to get adapted to pushing themselves for miles, so you're in for a doozy of an adaptation period. Keep your eye on the prize, and don't push yourself too far too fast or you'll get discouraged. When first beginning, try to get your heart rate at half your maximum and maintain your activity for only about 20 minutes. If you feel any joint pain, that's a sure sign to slow down. Remember that proper form is extremely important with any athletic movement, not just weightlifting, so really set those patterns of movement in your head to avoid injury and be on the path to look and feel your best.

Keto and supplementation

Any athlete worth his salt will tell you that half the fun of being active is the freedom to experiment on yourself like a mad scientist with all manner bizarre supplements, from creatine to the 57 varieties of protein powder in all of its artificial-tasting flavors. People on the keto diet may be in need of a few supplements to stay in good health, and it's important to know which common workout supplements it conflicts with and any adjustments you can make to keep taking it.

For staying healthy

This section should be proceeded with the disclaimer that supplements are not essential; that's why they're called supplements. Supplements should only be used when you need them, which, admittedly, can be hard to tell when. Keeping that in mind, some are "more" essential than others; almost all of us could use more omega-3s in our diet, for instance, and there's a good chance anyone on keto will need some electrolytes. It's perfectly possible to go on a keto diet and take no outside supplementation; it just requires an attention to detail above and beyond the usual.

- ☒ **Electrolytes**; potassium, sodium, and magnesium: Being low in any of these can make you feel like a dead man walking, and are indirectly the cause of many of the most awful keto flu symptoms - general irritation, insomnia, and muscle cramps and spasm. A little side effect of ketosis in its opening stages that a lot of people don't realize is your kidneys will be flushing you of water because of the lack of carbs, making you lose a lot of these salts in the process.

Sodium is important for proper firing of nerves and contracting of muscles. It's pretty easy to supplement this, literally just add salt to your foods. If your blood pressure is a problem, make sure not to overdo it and keep an eye on it in relation to your salt consumption.

Potassium: The first thing to know about potassium supplementation is this: Don't do it. Potassium can bleed over from the "Helps you stay alive" to "helps you stay dead" very quickly. The second thing to know is why you need it; it keeps your muscles from cramping, keeps your blood pressure steady, and is absolutely vital to keeping your heart pumping. Foods high in potassium are nuts, wild fish, and spinach, brussels sprouts, and avocado.

Magnesium: How do you figure you might be deficient in magnesium? Well, if you exist in America, that might a risk factor, as half of us are deficient. You'll also know if you have muscle cramps and spasms and problems sleeping. Men and women need anywhere from between 200 to 400 mg a day.

Calcium: Vital for muscle contractions which are necessary for everything. You'll need about 1,000 mg a day, and you can find it easily in things like whole canned fish fillets (bones and all!), yogurt and cheese, or supplementation.

- **Vitamin D:** One of the reasons vitamin D is important is that without it, calcium can't be absorbed, which can lead to further effects down the road in terms of muscular issues like weakness and fatigue. In addition, it's also vital for testosterone production. A good, cheap source is found right alongside calcium in canned bone-in sardines and for the more bourgeoisie amongst us (Or those who don't want sardine breath) fatty fresh fish.

- **Medium-Chain Triglyceride Oil, or MCT Oil:** MCT oil can function as what amounts to a cheat code for ketogenic dieters. They're immediately broken down into and shoved into the bloodstream where they can be used as ketones, and are a tasteless liquid fat that you can dump on everything you eat to make you feel full and keep you in ketosis.

- **Omega-3 Fatty Acids/Fish Oil:** There's been a lot of hubbub revolving around omega-3s in the last few years. They've been linked to improved brain health, cleansing of the arteries with lower triglyceride and higher HDL count, and reducing joint inflammation. It's fairly cheap for a giant container of them, but there are often questions about the quality of it and the potential for things like mercury or denatured acids so consider splurging. There's also some research suggesting it may be easier to absorb omega-3s in food forms, especially fish. If you don't want to break the bank and love sardines (we keep coming back to them don't we?) and fatty fish, they're a delicious, cheap, (In the case of sardines, anyway) and reliable way to get them in your diet.

- **Digestive enzymes:** Here's a strange-sounding one, but bear with me. When eating a diet higher in fat and protein than they're used to, it's not unusual that people can report some gastric symptoms and might need a little outside help until they're adapted, so they don't experience those feelings we all know and love; bloating, nausea, and vomiting. Supplemental digestive enzymes can help with these symptoms as they're literally the things your body makes to digest food but in pill form.

- ☒ **Exogenous ketones**: Ketones made outside the body, as the name suggests. They can help you stay in ketosis if you haven't measured your carb intake correctly, and potentially even induce a state of deeper ketosis. The best exogenous ketones are made from the best, most efficient endogenous ketones - look for a variety composed mostly of beta-hydroxybutyrate.
- ☒ **Green Powder:** Something I wish was an option when I was a kid. Dried, powdered greens, maybe the same kind of stuff they use to turn the spinach pasta green. But it's the perfect supplement who can't seem to jam in enough vegetables to their diet, which isn't surprising given their main macronutrient composition is carbohydrates.

Common workout supplements and keto

Athletes take all manner of interesting-sounding lab creations to get in shape, from creatine to BCAAs to whey powder. Do they mesh with keto? Some do, some don't. When picking a workout supplement, avoid the ones with added sugar, this mostly applies to pre-workout drinks and protein powders. While the science of the dangers of artificial sweeteners is up in the air, it's generally a good idea to forsake those too when you can. There are so many supplements that they can't all be covered here, especially the illegal ones, but a good rule of thumb is that if there's no sugar, you're good to go.

- ☒ **BCAAs** - Branched-chain amino acids. Not really necessary, as long as you eat enough protein. Most people who go on keto end up eating more protein anyway, so this shouldn't be necessary, but doesn't necessarily harm you.

- ☒ **Protein** - Pea, collagen, soy, whey protein, there are a million varieties, and they all have minute differences. Protein supplements work fine with keto as long as you're keeping your fat in higher percentages, and there's little to no added sugar.

- ☒ **Creatine** - One of the more infamous supplements in the world of athletics, despite it being possibly one of the most effective. Creatine supplements are used to power the creatine phosphate system, and there are serious links between its usage and improved athletic ability. Creatine and ketosis get along fine and share tea like civilized people as long as creatine contains no added sugar.

- ☒ **Taurine** – Taurine has come on to the stage in recent years because of its ability to patch a hole in ketosis' weakest point, energy system wise. It's been shown to improve anaerobic ability and reduce fatigue. Taurine has a stamp of approval for ketosis as well because it's great for what ketosis is bad at and contains no carbs.

- ☒ **Caffeine** – Caffeine is a double-edged sword on ketosis. It can raise cortisol levels, which is bad for ketosis. But, at the same time, it's fantastic for suppressing appetite, especially when blended with some coconut oil or butter, making a useful tool for weight loss. Also, there have been real, demonstrable effects that show that caffeine improves cardiovascular endurance. Whether or not caffeine is right for you is a personal question, many people can't function without it, and the increased cortisol levels aren't a problem. In fact, one of the infamous keto trends that have bled into wider society is "bulletproof coffee," the aforementioned coffee and butter, coffee and coconut oil, or for the truly daring, coffee and lard.

☒ **L-Citrulline** - Coming from the Latin word for "watermelon," citrulline helps promote blood flow in the body by way of obnoxiously complex biochemistry. It can lead to better pumps for bodybuilders as well as increased aerobic and anaerobic performance and would be ideal for the bodybuilder still adapting to his new diet.

Keto and exercise: A lot to consider

Exercise takes everything you know about resting metabolic rate and effectively makes it 5 times more complicated, displayed neatly by the length of this chapter. It's really impossible to know if ketosis and exercise walk hand-in-hand sweetly without knowing a lot more about exercise physiology and the types of activities themselves, which this chapter set out to illuminate. Hopefully, with this chapter ingrained into the mind and a fair bit of rumination on gripping topics like the phosphagen energy system, steady state cardio, and what supplements to take to avoid dropping like a fly after a workout, the right decision for your particular exercise wants and needs can be made.

Chapter 9: Keto While Vegan

Ketosis and a vegan diet is a tricky balancing act that is not accomplished by merely drinking coconut oil and crying. Vegan diets, as a refresher, are a diet free of all animal products, no meat, fish, eggs, dairy, or honey. They can be challenging to stick to on their own, much less trying to accomplish on keto, given that animal products tend to be more rich in fat and protein. Alas, it's not an entirely insurmountable task with enough nutritional knowledge and a fair bit of cooking tricks and tips.

For a vegan to go keto and keep their constitution, it's important that they know their healthiest options for fat and protein. Generally speaking, avocados, MCT oil, coconuts and coconut oil, fatty tofu (A thing I didn't know existed until I did my research for this chapter) and possibly the vegan's most powerful ally, nutritional yeast, especially the kind fortified with B12, will be your best friends. A keto vegan diet isn't going to be vastly different in terms of nutrient content than a regular keto diet, just very restrictive with what you can eat.

Cover your bases

Protein

Hopefully, dear reader, you are prepared for another long ramble on biochemistry, as without the knowledge you'd be scratching your head wondering why a vegan can't just eat 100 grams of seitan (extracted wheat gluten; also technically the "most" protein dense food) and call it a day. Well, the reason is because of amino acids. They are what makes up the delicious protein in all living things, and there are 20 of them. Eleven of these acids the body can make on its own, but there are nine it can't, which we need to get from food. All animal products containing protein have all nine in them wrapped up in a neat little bow, but not all plants do. In fact, there is a serious dearth of plant products that contain all nine amino acids we need, but thankfully this can be remedied by eating two kinds of plant protein together. The classic example is beans and rice, which has probably kept more people healthy than all medicine in all time ever.

Unfortunately, when going on a ketogenic diet, beans and rice aren't really an option, because while they combine to make a complete protein that the body can use for muscle growth and maintenance, they also contain a much higher percentage of carbohydrates, far too much to go ketogenic on. There are complete sources of protein, such as quinoa and buckwheat are personal favorites. The problem here is twofold; neither are super common in the western diet, so it helps to have a culinary flair to make them more appreciable, but this ignores the elephant in the room. The bigger problem is the fact that quinoa and buckwheat have served as staple crops for peoples in South America and Eastern Europe, respectively, for generations. Staple crops are, by nature, always energy-rich, they're high carbohydrate foods and therefore are not compatible with going keto.

Before really getting into the "meat" of it (heh), a special note should be made amount vegan "meats," as while they tend to be full of complete protein, many of them contain added carbohydrates and potentially unsavory additives, so it's important to check the ingredient list and nutritional content. Make sure the fat and protein are as close to normal meat as you can find, and that all the ingredients are things that you could potentially get right in a spelling bee. Nuts are also lauded as a source of protein, and while they are, oftentimes eating a lot of them can result in going over carbohydrate count, and they are not usually "complete" sources of protein.

Tofu and tempeh are two sides of the same coin, both are made from soybeans, and both are known for being bland and hard to get used to. Tempeh wins in that category because it's famous for being "bland, grainy, and slightly bitter," but with enough cooking knowledge, they are capable of amazing things, as they drink up the taste of whatever you cook with them, and are an excellent addition to soups and stews.

Nutritional yeast is also a criminally underrepresented vegan protein source. It has only one gram of net carb from carbohydrate, four grams of fiber, and nine grams of complete protein and a lot of it is fortified already with B12. It's the deactivated cousin of the fungal friend of humanity's that helps us make bread and has a taste that is weirdly reminiscent of cheese, so it's great for the former cheesemonger turned vegan.

Lastly, if fungi-dressed-up-as-cheese nor soy products are your thing, there's a third option for covering protein, but it's not "food" per se. Pea protein powder is a widely available supplement, and a complete protein to boot. So if you're having a hard time keeping the yeast and soy down, a pea protein shake mixed with MCTs might be just the thing.

Fat

For fat, you can be thankful that many vegan sources are unambiguously healthy -as long as they're minimally processed, and there are plenty of them, making getting your daily fat requirement simple. Olives, avocados, coconuts, nuts, and seeds in their various forms, and the oils extracted from them.

For saturated fat, the best (and most ethical) vegan source are coconuts and its oil. The reason "most ethical" is a point of contention is twofold – one is the inherent fact that many vegans are very concerned with ethics, given the nature of their diet. The other point is that palm oil production is infamously destructive in the area where it's typically farmed; southeastern Asia.

When cooking with fat, it's important to know the smoke point of your oils, if oil smokes, it's going toxic and producing free radicals, not something you want to be putting into your body. Non-vegans have a little more free reign with this, as they have access to fats like ghee, lard, and tallow, but given the veganism's restrictive nature, knowing how to cook with limited options is extremely important. Avocado oil is the shining star, having the highest heat amongst all cooking oils at 520 degrees Fahrenheit. So if you're deep frying some tofu fritters (is that a thing?) this would be the optimal choice. If you're looking to do lower-heat cooking, say sautéing garlic and onions before adding it to a sauce, virgin, unrefined olive or coconut oil is your better choice. These oils have a more delicate flavor and lower smoke point, so keeping them below that keeps its unique taste as well as keeping free radicals from causing a ruckus in your system.

Micronutrients and their buddies

A vegan keto diet might also be low in a number of other micronutrients, all of which can be found in the form of an appetizing supplemental capsule.

- ☒ Vitamin D: While it can be acquired from lightly toasting yourself by the pool, there are better ways of getting it. Namely, supplementation, but trace amounts can be found in mushrooms.

- ☒ Vitamin B12: This is another big hole in the vegan diet; because it can only come from animal sources and certain microorganisms. Many vegan foods are fortified with it, but it's also available in capsule form as well. Vitamin B12 necessary for proper digestion of fats and proteins, development of the myelin sheath that coats your neurons, and erythrogenesis; the production of red blood cells. It's important to say that there are some vitamin and mineral deficiencies that you can suffer through. Obviously they should be treated, but they don't hit you as hard as B12 deficiency, because B12 deficiency WILL kill you much faster.

- Vitamin C: You figure a vegan would have plenty of options to vitamin C, right? It's mainly found in plant sources, so there should be no trouble. Well, vitamin C is a delicate flower that is easily annihilated by heat and found a lot in fruit. And guess what you'll be eating as a vegan on keto? Not a lot of fruit and probably a lot of cooked vegetables. It's pretty easy to get this in the form of raw vegetables, most notably bell peppers and certain cruciferous vegetables; broccoli, cabbage, kale, and brussels sprouts.

- Calcium: Here's a big one; calcium is vital for bone strength and keeping the heart working. it's found easily in a number of animal products; dairy, cold water fatty fish, even eggshells if you're that much of an eccentric. If you're low on it, it's found in a variety of nuts and seeds, like sesame and tahini (tahini is a paste made from sesame seeds and oil) and flaxseed, and of course, in pill form.

- Zinc: This one is big for the boys, as it's essential for testosterone, but also for fighting off infection. It's somewhat more difficult to drain it from plant-based sources, so you may have to eat more to get the same amount. Again, it's found in nuts and seeds like sesame and tahini, pumpkin and sunflower seeds, and cashews. There's a trend here.

- ⊠ Iron: Unless you like slipping into anemia, you need this. Again, it's harder to absorb non-heme (plant) iron than heme (animal) iron, so eat more than usual. Men are recommended to have 8, women 18 mg a day, but when you go vegan, it's closer to 12 and 33 a day. Common sources are spinach, olives, and tahini, sesame, chia, and pumpkin seeds.

- ⊠ Omega-3s: One of the magic pills of the modern diet, and for most people comes from the oils of fish. Flaxseed oil and flaxseed oil tablets might be the thing to rush to, but they contain less EPA and DHA, which contain most of the more lauded health benefits of the omega-3 family. APA is in much higher quantities, but at the same time is not really the one that yields any health benefits. Instead, your body converts it to EPA and DHA. And very inefficiently, I might add. So, to get your fill of these two important fatty acids, consider seaweed/algae. It is indirectly the source of the omega-3s in fish, so go straight to the source and get it where the sardines get it.

Vegan substitutions

So you want to go vegan, but aren't willing to start eating entirely akin to your herbivorous friends in the woods; nuts, seeds, and greens, and don't want to be making a paste of coconut oil and nutritional yeast like those of us in civilization, you'd like to keep your diet as close to "normal" as possible. Fear not, for the answer lies here. Many common foods that are not vegan have vegan replacement options to make transitioning just a little easier.

Milk

Milk is where both keto and vegans can proudly raise their banner, because it's not great for ketosis, given the carbohydrate count, and completely incompatible with veganism. There are a number of options to consider, and if buying them premade, remember to get the kind with no added sugars.

Coconut milk derives almost 100% of its calories from fat, a small amount of carbs and protein. It's a great source of medium chain triglycerides, which, if you remember, are often bottled and sold as a supplement as they are more easily used as energy than other forms of triglycerides.

Almond milk is the second runner up, with a higher ratio of carbs to fat, somewhere around 1:3, so for every gram of carb you get three of fat. It's relatively easy to make at home and packed with micronutrients, and it doesn't go under as much processing as soy milk, with the added benefit of there being no chance for it to screw with your hormones, and this applies to both men and women, as soy contains phytoestrogens.

Pea milk is another potential player, it contains an identical amount of protein as dairy milk, and tastes nothing like the mushy green orbs of deliciousness you may hate/love. The reason is that it's made from a flour that is then mixed with water and oil, keeping your protein and fat needs satisfied without throwing you into a bind with excess carbs.

Butter

When it comes to keto and vegan butter, there is really only one-stand in, and that's virgin coconut oil. It's spreadable and saturated just the same way, and is near identical in terms of fat content.

Yogurt

Yogurt is what happens when you introduce a certain bacteria in a certain liquid at a certain temperature and let it sit overnight, which is why there are perfectly viable options made from coconut, cashew, and almond that a ketogenic vegan can enjoy, so as long as there are no added sugars.

Cheese and cream cheese

There are a number of non-dairy cheeses made from tree nuts and soy. The best mimic for the taste of cheese, if not the texture, I retain to be nutritional yeast. Cream cheese substitutes can be made at home using cashews, but watch out for sugar content.

Eggs

Ground flaxseed - The most common substitute for eggs, when it comes to baking at least, is ground flaxseed mixed with water. If you've ever eaten whole flax seed, there's an almost waxy, gooey bit that forms as you pulverize it with your teeth. When you mix one tablespoon of flax with three of water, it serves the same binding purpose an egg does, imparting no flavor, merely serving in the same "structural" role. Chia seeds will also work for this, used in the same way with the same ratio.

Baking soda and vinegar - Two delicious stand-ins for eggs when you need to make something fluffier, which flaxseed is woefully under-equipped to do. The reaction they form makes whatever you're cooking bubbly and more airy. One teaspoon of baking soda to a tablespoon of vinegar is the usual ratio.

Silken Tofu does the opposite of baking soda and vinegar and is great for making foods denser than a neutron star. Like all tofu, it tastes like a glass of water would taste if you removed the flavor, so it's inoffensive and smoother than other tofu varieties. ¼ of a cup of it is about an egg.

The last thing to say is that there are a variety of premade egg substitutes on the market, and if you're considering them, remember to check the ingredients and nutritional value. The fat and protein ratio of both these premade substitutes and the ones you make in your kitchen will obviously not match that of a real egg, so keep your macronutrients in mind when using them.

Going back to our roots

While going keto and being vegan may seem difficult at first, with the right knowledge and a mind willing to experiment in the kitchen, it's easily attainable. Keep your diet rich in protein sources like tofu, nutritional yeast, and pea protein, eat plenty of healthy fats and remember to patch any holes in your dietary armor with any number of supplements. And keep your head up when trying to create the perfect egg or yogurt substitute, this part requires a bit of experimentation, and it's easy to get discouraged. "Fall down seven times, get up eight."

Chapter 10: Keto Myths

Keto myths are, unfortunately, nothing as colorful and hilarious as something like the mystical 13th labor of Hercules, where, using a keto diet, he shredded the excess fat from all the wine and bread to beat Thor for the first time in the Mr. Divinity contest; nor are they as backwoodsy as the legendary Florida Keto Ape, who breaks into your home, rifles through your pantry and steals all your MCTs and expensive olive oil. No, unfortunately, keto myths are more along the lines of "can too much protein at once kick me out of ketosis?" and "Can I go into ketoacidosis and die a horrible death?" Much, much drier, and require a lot more breakdown than the legend that the soma drank by Indo-Iranics was actually MCT oil. There is any number of different myths surrounding keto, but in this chapter, we'll try to cover some of the more conventional ones, the problems, and questions that are more likely to sew doubt in your mind.

1. Too much protein at once can kick me out of ketosis

We've started with one of the hardest ones, and it's tempting to believe, as your body uses the constituents of proteins, amino acids, along with a slew of other organic compounds to form glucose in the body. It's not as cut and dry as a yes or no, because the answer is closer to "no, but maybe yes. Depends on you man." To be frank, in both diabetics and nondiabetics, protein does not turn to sugar in any noticeable quantity, BUT it will spike insulin and glucagon. How much spikes your insulin depends on a number of factors - which is why the answer is GENERALLY "No if you're a healthy, non-diabetic adult," but everyone is different, so it's important that you learn how much protein you need. We'll cover the methodology of testing before we go into the why. This entire book, I've been praising 20% as the usual percentage, but that can be more or less, depending on you. This is one of the reasons why measuring your ketones is so bloody important.

Speaking of blood, a blood test strip is the best way to find your optimal protein requirement. Go on the keto diet for a week, keep your carbs at 5% and your protein at 20% and your fat at 75% of your daily intake. This should be enough to put you in ketosis. Then, test yourself. If you fall below 1.5 mmol/L, decrease your protein count by 5% and increase fat by 5% and test yourself again a week later. Repeat as needed and adjust your protein consumption accordingly.

Your protein need depends on a lot of things, to keep it short and sweet, men, especially active men need more. Your body composition matters, more muscular people will need more, and if you're trying to put on muscle, you'll need more. If you've been on keto a long time as well, your body is more used to using ketones, so the protein you consume is less likely to spike insulin to any degree. Lastly, there are factors outside your control that will determine protein consumption; namely genetics and insulin sensitivity. The more insulin sensitive you are, the less it interferes, and vice-versa.

2. You can go keto one day and go off it the next

Yo-yo dieting is one of the many characters in a metabolic rogue's gallery that our bodies just cannot tolerate. It leads to increased weight gain, increased risk of diabetes, and increased mortality. The jump from fat to skinny causes more stress on you than just carrying the extra weight. In the ketogenic diet, this is manifested in the person who eats keto one day and then carbohydrates the next and then back to keto the next day, forever and ever, ad infinitum. This is NOT how the keto diet works. The keto diet does best when the body adapts to it over time. The more adapted you are, the more efficient it gets at keeping off your weight, it burns more ketones, your brain gets more fed, everything gets more efficient. When you jump on and off it, you're basically putting your body through indecisive metabolic trauma and not getting the benefits of eating one way or the other. You might be going through symptoms of keto flu every time you try it for a day.

3. Ketosis is free reign to stuff your craw with deep-fried butter and pork belly

Everything in moderation is a life maxim that applies almost everywhere, almost. Obviously, you won't be eating a modest amount of carbohydrates, but that's not the point. Saturated fat, the solid-at-room-temperature fat that characterizes the fat in animal products, is good for you, good for hormones, HDLs, IN APPROPRIATE AMOUNTS. It's easy to go overboard with saturated fat because it's so delicious, and so many sources of fat are animal products. But the keto diet celebrates all fat, and monounsaturated fats are the unambiguous stars of health in the fat world. Enjoy a steak, enjoy salmon, butter, or lard, but keep it in moderation with plenty of healthy fats as well, because too much-saturated fat can lead to arterial clogging. If it's economically permissible, getting meat from locally sourced, humanely-treated animals and wild fish and game will always carry additional benefits.

4. Nutrient proportions are set in stone

No one can blame you if you read this book and think that I'm espousing that line of thinking, as I have continuously come back to the percentage of 75%–20%–5% of fat, protein, and carbs, over and over again. The first myth talked about particular protein requirements, as you can see, everyone is different. This also applies to carbohydrates, fats, and micronutrients. Some of us just don't need as much as others, or some of us need more. Say you're three or four weeks into the keto diet, you've tested yourself, and you're in deep ketosis, and, to top it all off, let's even say you're being a good little ketogenic and consuming MCTs. If you still feel like a hardboiled egg thrown across a greasy windshield (And do let me know how that feels) and your ketone levels are in the optimal range, and you're eating, say, 20 grams of carbs a day, it's perfectly possible that you're not getting enough of them. Up your carbohydrate intake by 10 grams or so and see how you feel, but remember to keep testing yourself and not go over the new limit you've set.

5. Ketosis is a risk factor for ketoacidosis

While it's true that your body has to enter ketosis before it goes into ketoacidosis, that doesn't mean that ketoacidosis is the logical conclusion to ketosis. Ketoacidosis is when your blood ketones rise so high you're in potentially life-threatening levels, which is a risk factor for those with diabetes mellitus, not ketogenic dieters, it's simply not a risk factor.

6. Ketosis is the ultimate, final way to lose weight

Though there are thousands of books claiming this, this isn't even close to true. Keto is a diet, and every diet doesn't work for everybody. Genetic conditions exist that make it hard for people's bodies to access and use the stored fat they have as fuel; others may simply not feel like following such a strict program. There are also risk factors if you do it wrong, muscle wasting, an increased psychological deviation that can lead to binge eating of unhealthy foods, which is why it's not the best long term solution for all of us, even most of us. It requires a certain discipline to make it work, for most of us it's a short-term solution that may work wonderfully when we're injured or don't have access to the gym for whatever reason. There's only one real "final" diet concept to swallow in case you need to drop weight, and that's calorie counting. If you can make sure that the calories you take in are less than those that you spend, you will lose weight. The problem with that is that it won't necessarily be the way you want, and it may be even more difficult for some of us than ketogenic dieting. Really, it's that, or to stop eating entirely.

7. Ketosis is a high protein diet

Let's get one thing cleared up; ketosis is a diet higher in protein than most people are probably used to because a lot more of our calories will be coming from animal products, which are high in protein. Having eggs and ham for breakfast and a steak for dinner may be the right kind of food for ketosis, but too much without tempering it with fat will simply cause the diet to fail and your ketosis to never occur. In addition, the chance of slipping into ketoacidosis for non-diabetics is very low; the chance increases if you eat too much protein when you're in deep ketosis. Amino acid breakdown into your blood could-potentially-maybe-might-possibly increase them even more, putting your blood at dangerously acidic levels.

8. Ketosis destroys your heart and valves

This is an easy one to see, because of the stark increase in fat and animal protein that people usually consume, but it's simply unfounded. When used correctly and weight is lost, as to what happens to those who follow the diet correctly, it lowers risk of heart disease. Furthermore, as long as you aren't consuming pork lard coated with butter, your triglyceride and LDL count should stay the same. Numerous studies have shown that low carb dieters versus low-fat dieters have had lower blood cholesterol and that the diet can effectively raise the HDL, "good" cholesterol, and improve signs like blood pressure.

9. Keto can cause flu-like symptoms

By now, you should be familiar with this one. This one is technically true, but only in the short-term adaptation period. Once there are a sufficient number of ketones in the bloodstream, and your brain has accepted them as its new fuel source, the fog should be lifted, and you'll be back to your old self.

10. Ketosis exacerbates fatty liver

If you can recall earlier in the book, one of the benefits of ketosis is that it has the power to loosen in particular the tough-to-get-at, really deep in, abdominal fat. Well, guess where the liver is? If you guessed the abdomen, I have good news! With this line of reasoning, we can pretty safely assume that the diet will do a fantastic job at helping alleviate fatty liver rather than making it worse. In fact, diets high in carbohydrates and alcohol are really the culprit in making it worse.

11. Ketosis carries out a systematic extermination of your gut flora

The source of this claim usually has something to do with the fact that certain keto-gone-wrong diets can be low in fiber, which wreaks havoc on everything stomach and below. In a well-balanced ketogenic diet, you should be getting tons of fiber, as though fiber is a carb, it's not digestible and therefore has no effect on blood sugar. If you're doing it right, you'll be eating plenty of fibrous vegetables. Some studies have shown that a ketogenic diet done right can be beneficial for gut flora, as carbohydrates can nourish some of the negative strains.

12. Any fat is good fat

The majority of the fat you should consume on the keto diet should be monounsaturated fat and a smaller amount of saturated fat, optimally from healthy, happy animals and wild fish. Putting a lot of polyunsaturated, highly processed corn, soybean, and vegetable oils is a waste of calories but not necessarily awful. There's no additional nutrients, and aren't high in MCTs, but good for hitting your macros if nothing else shows itself. It's also not an excuse to eat fast food hamburgers with no bun, because if the suspicious meat that doesn't decay after a year wasn't enough to keep you away, being cooked in artery-destroying trans-fat will.

And so it is written

The mythology surrounding the ketogenic diet is not like the exciting stories of the Theogony or Aeneid, and nowhere near as personally inspiring

(For most people, I'd estimate) but they are far more harmful and far more applicable in daily life. They spread misinformation about the diet, which can have a serious effect on those people who it might help who are looking to try it. For every person scared away by false knowledge, that's a person the keto diet could have helped.

Chapter 11: Good Foods

While theoretically you could approach keto and eat nothing but protein and greens powder mixed with water and washed down with olive and coconut oil, that is by far the worst and possibly silliest way to go about it. This chapter is dedicated to the best whole foods you can eat on keto, and those to avoid. It's not attempting to be a comprehensive or exhaustive list, but more as a guide to light your way and set you upon the path.

Fats and oils

- Extra-virgin olive oil - A strong tasting monounsaturated fat. Has serious benefits for reducing LDLs, blood pressure improves skin quality and could help with depression, Alzheimer's.

- Virgin coconut oil - In its refined form, saturated but still very healthy. It's full of MCTs, which are quickly tossed into the metabolic furnace as fuel, and has been connected with lower rates of inflammation.

- Avocado oil - Possibly the best oil for frying, as it has a 520-degree Fahrenheit smoke point. Monounsaturated, with a similar oleic acid content as extra virgin olive oil, giving it pro-cardiac, LDL lowering potencies.

- ☒ Lard - Not deserving of its reputation as an artery-clogging cardiac nightmare, from the right pigs and rendered from scraps at home, lard can be high in monounsaturated fat and full of omega-3s

- ☒ Grass-fed butter and ghee - Keyword here is grass-fed. Grass-fed steps all over grain-fed health wise - more vitamins, conjugated linoleic acid, and omega-3s. In case you aren't a nutritionist, know that conjugated linoleic acid has a smorgasbord of random health benefits, supporting bone health, muscle development, and soothing inflammation. And what is ghee, you may ask? Well, I'm glad you asked. Ghee is clarified butter - butter with the milk solids strained out, with a similar nutrient profile and fantastic for high-heat cooking.

Meat, poultry, and seafood

- ☒ Fatty fish - You want to go heavy on the fish that looks like it can't fit into its pants anymore, but keep it wild. Wild, fatty fish - think salmon, trout, sardines, kippers, herring, and tuna, is the most famous and abundant source of omega-3s we know of, along with high-quality fat and protein. Omega-3s curb inflammation, contribute to brain and heart health and keep the eyeballs working. They also contain large amounts of vitamin D, and, if canned fish is your thing, calcium from the bones. If you're concerned about mercury content, go small with tiny canned fish. Because they are the wimps of the ocean and are low on the food chain, they don't contain huge chunks of mercury (as a way of speaking) like the bigger fish, such as tuna.

- ☒ Grass-fed beef/local beef - Depends if you want to get up early enough in the morning to go to your local farmer's market. Grass-fed beef contains higher amounts of omega-3s, vitamin B and E, beta-carotene, and conjugated linoleic acid than corn-fed beef. It also contains less fat - to make up for that, choose the fattier cuts like rib or chuck cuts. Local beef depends on your farmer, but usually small-time farmers have healthier, happier animals who pass this benefit up to you. Talk to your local farmer and see what he feeds his cows to get a better idea of what you're getting.

- ☒ Pasture-raised pork: There's a trend amongst meat; and that's when the animal is happier and healthier, it comes out tasting better and better for you — what a strange idea. Not only does their meat have a better flavor with a higher fat content than factory raised pork, but their fat is also rich in vitamin D, and omega-3s and their meat isn't contaminated with antibiotics and growth hormone.

- ☒ Pasture-raised chicken: Consider buying dark meat, as it's more nutritious, higher in fat, and cheaper. Like the other humanely-raised meat, pasture-raised chicken is higher in omega-3s and lower in omega-6s, with higher counts of selenium and B3 than its conventional, factory farmed cousin. B3 is important for energy and digestion, and selenium is a potent antioxidant.

- ☒ Pasture-raised eggs: The spawn of pasture-raised chickens, and most definitely a meat despite people trying to categorize them as "dairy." Eggs have been called "nature's perfect food," and it's not hard to see why. They come prepackaged with a durable outer container, a great percentage of fat and protein can be used in nearly everything, and it's easy to eat five or six of them without feeling like death. Not being raised in what can be described as a hellish dungeon for chickens, pasture-raised eggs have oodles more omega-3 and vitamin E than their prison-spawned equivalents.

☒ Bone broth: Not technically a meat, but what happens when you suspend gelatin, protein, and fat in water. The collagen has great benefits for your skin, nails, and joints, and make sure to add plenty of salt for both electrolytes and to make it taste less like a barnyard.

A note on meat and seafood: Almost any pasture-raised, humanely slaughtered meat is going to be good on the ketogenic diet, but it's not a necessity. It can get expensive quickly, especially if you're an athlete. In that case, consider supplements for the micronutrients and omega-3s you'll be missing. In addition, other meats, such as mutton and lamb, chevron (goat meat), offal, and veal are all fantastic choices when eaten in the right proportions. You may have noticed that shellfish was omitted - it appears shellfish is slightly higher in carbohydrates, depending on the type eaten, than other kinds of seafood, which is why it can't be recommended in earnest as a great food. It can, of course, be a part of a healthy ketogenic diet, as long as you make sure that you limit how much of it you eat.

Nuts, Seeds, Legumes, etc.:

There's not really an easy category for these guys, so they go alone. They contain everything in your mixed nuts jar - peanuts, almonds, sesame, sunflower seeds, so on and so forth. All of them can be made into jars of butter at home with a blender and some grit. All of them are rich sources of monounsaturated fat, fiber, and protein, so, in a quest to not repeat myself too often, only the micronutrient profiles and other benefits will be highlighted. Also, not all of them will be listed, because that would take probably way more space than necessary, only the more common specimens.

- Peanuts: Minerals like copper and manganese
- Almonds: Biotin and vitamin E
- Sunflower seeds: A combination of the two lads above them, rich in Vitamin E and copper.
- Walnuts: When consumed skin on, flavonoids and other antioxidants. Omega-3s and copper are found in the flesh of the walnut.
- Sesame: Omega-3s, copper, and manganese, which is why it was often referred to as the "eastern peanut." The last part is made up.

There are obviously hundreds of breeds of nuts in existence, and it would be akin to Sisyphus and his boulder to list them all, but in general, nuts are a fantastic source of nutrition for the keto dieter and a worthy addition to their nutritional arsenal for both snacking and cooking.

Fruits:

Most fruit is right out because of its high sugar content, but there are two "stars."

- ☒ Avocado: If you didn't see this coming, you might need to make sure you can actually read. Avocado has so many health benefits the rest of this chapter could be dedicated to it, but I'll resist and give a basic overview. Avocados are full of fiber and monounsaturated fat, vitamins K, C, B, and E, and tons of potassium. They're also filling, VERY self-contained, and versatile. Delicious in protein shakes!

- ☒ Olives: Olives have a very similar nutritional content to olive oil. Who'd have thought it? Monounsaturated fat, antioxidants, and vitamin E come pre-packed in a nice little orb. If you're watching the sodium intake putting a hard limit on them isn't such an unwise idea.

Vegetables:

In this context, vegetables in fruit are sort of opposite. Low carb vegetables are absolute darlings, and eat as many as you can in as many varieties as you can. Because most vegetables are inherently low carb and good for you, we're going to have a similar policy and pick only a handful of true standouts. If there's something not on the list here and your body desires of it, look up the nutritional information to assure it fits your carb goals, and enjoy. It will be said here and nowhere else that every single vegetable is full of fiber, so I don't sound like a broken record.

- ☒ Tomatoes: Not only are they good for throwing at bad stage actors, but fresh tomatoes are also delicious raw, cooked, or in a sauce or soup. Look to our red friends for micronutrients like vitamins C and K, (vitamin C when raw) potassium, and B9, the experimental sci-fi name for folate.

- ☒ Brassica family vegetables: Hold your horses, before you start throwing whole cabbages at me, think of this as an experiment in efficiency. ALL brassica (cabbage) family veggies are good for you. This includes cabbage (wow!) cabbagini (a custom word that means "small cabbage" - brussels sprout) broccoli, kale, and cauliflower. All of these veggies are chock full of antioxidants, vitamin C, vitamin K, potassium, and iron. A word of warning - there's a chance in poisoning yourself if you eat too much kale from the huge bomb of vitamin K. As a way to enjoy these foods that typically might make adults and children cringe, try serving them up with a huge scoop of butter or bacon. Really eases the bitterness.

- ☒ Spinach: Obligatory Popeye, the Sailor Man joke, followed up with actual nutritional information. Famed for its iron and ability to spontaneously generate massive amounts of muscular power in nautical tough guys, it also has plenty of folic acids, calcium, and phytonutrients. If you're anything like me, you'll be tempted to knock on your dentist's door and ask him why your teeth are failing because of the weird grittiness on your teeth. That's a certain type of acid found in broken down spinach - not harmful, but if it's in a bad mood it might stop you from absorbing some of that iron, so give it a spritz of lemon or lime juice before you uppercut Brutus into the stratosphere.

- ☒ Eggplant: Eggplant is interesting, it's not necessarily packed with any nutrients besides the obligatory fiber and medium dose of manganese, and it should be salted an hour before consumed because of a compound related to nicotine makes it taste bitter, but it's a potentially powerful tool for keeping you full. The reason being is that it drinks up the flavors of whatever you cook it in, so it could be filled with nutritious and filling olive oil and tomato sauce or whatever else you choose to be its vessel.

- ☒ Asparagus: If there's any vegetable best suited for pretending you're in an ancient Greek phalanx wielding a *dory* (spear) at the dinner table, it's asparagus. Besides for LARPing, asparagus is useful for being filled with vitamins A, C, E, and K. And as easily as the Hellenic *dory* fends off Persian armies and reduces near-eastern influence, asparagus' high antioxidant content fends off free radicals and reduces oxidative stress.

Dairy

The big kid on campus of dairy, milk, is technically acceptable, but probably not the best choice as it does have quite a bit of sugar per serving. The good news is that in two of its mutant forms, cheese, and yogurt, it's much lower in lactose but still full of protein, calcium, and vitamin D. If you haven't figured it out by now, go with the full-fat varieties, for reasons of satiety.

- ☒ Cheese: The enzymy, degenerate, delicious form of milk. It's filling and full of protein and healthy fat and almost no carbs. It's almost like a form of curdled meat product in terms of nutritional value - and contains calcium. Whole fat mozzarella cheese sticks are an excellent snack, roughly the equivalent of a boiled egg if you don't feel like boiling it and destroying half of it as you peel it.

- ☒ Yogurt: Here's a classic joke originating from the central Asian steppe, where yogurt originated: What do you get when you leave your milk in a leather pouch for too long? Yogurt! Obviously, these steppe nomads had a poorly developed sense of humor. Yogurt has a few more carbs but has the upside of being a probiotic food. As mentioned in the "joke" earlier, yogurt was found to have originated from old milk left in a leather pouch carried by steppe peoples, and was probably a cozy home for Lactobacillus, as it quickly migrated to the milk to form yogurt. The lactobacillus colonizes your gut, and can positively affect everything from muscular pain to mental health. As a rule, pick strained - or Greek - yogurt, as its higher in protein and lower and carbs. Much like mozzarella sticks, strained yogurt is usually sold prepackaged in containers with all of its nutritional information on the side.

- Heavy cream: Finally, our dreams of coffee half-cream half-coffee are realized. Heavy cream is great for meeting our fat goals and is a tasty addition to scores of dishes.
- Sour cream/Creme fraiche: For the Tex-Mex lovers, I have kept you from your beans, rice, and tortillas. But I have bestowed upon you the privilege of your delicious sour cream condiment, as it is essentially all fat. The same goes for creme fraiche, actually slightly higher in fat content than sour cream, and goes great with eggs.

Snacks:

- Pork rinds: Keto chips can take two forms, and one of them is a bit of deep-fried pork skin. Pork rinds are a great source of protein and fat, far more filling than regular potato chips, and can be made at home.
- Parmesan chips: The other form of the keto chip and possibly one of the tastiest culinary innovations in recent years. They have the same nutrition as parmesan/romano cheese, high in protein and fat, and are simple to make at home. Probably less of a time investment than the pork rinds, really.
- Dehydrated vegetables: If you own a dehydrator, rejoice. You can dry any number

of leafy greens and other vegetables in huge amounts and end up with much smaller amounts of snacks the next day. When made at home, you can customize their flavor however you want and are far cheaper than the ones made in the store. In addition, you can trust that there are no suspicious unpronounceable additives. Dehydrated vegetables retain all the nutrition of regular vegetables, as the low heat of dehydration isn't enough to denature them. They can also be done with an oven on the lowest setting and enough patience.

Drinks:

- ☒ Water: You will die in three days max without water. You are 70% water. That should be enough to get you to drink it. It's absolutely necessary for all life functions, it's refreshing, and keeps hunger at bay. If you need a little bit of extra flavor, try adding lemon, lime, grapefruit, or cucumber to your water and refrigerating it overnight.

- ☒ Tea and coffee: As long as they're unsweetened, you can have your caffeine. One of the keto rages is bulletproof coffee - I see no reason why the same idea can't theoretically work with tea as well. Try blending in a bit of butter into your tea if you're used to taking it with milk for an energy boost, and report back to me on how it tasted.

Foods to avoid, or at least eat in moderation:

Foods to avoid on this diet tends to be a little more apparent if you actually read this book. A general rule of good nutrition is to avoid processed foods, sugar, and trans fat. Keto takes all these rules and turns its furious gaze on starchy carbohydrates and fruit as well.

Fats:

- Polyunsaturated fat: These are fats like your typical cooking oils - corn oil, peanut oil, canola oil, and soybean oil. There's nothing particularly bad about these oils - they are heavily processed and contain less nutrients than monounsaturated fats like avocado, olive, or coconut oils. Their strongest upside is they're cheap. They technically are fine if you need your fat for the day, but there are much better choices, with more omega-3s and linoleic acid.

- Trans Fat: Now this guy is definitely a shady character. Trans fats are found in processed foods; fast food burgers, pizza, and all its other deviant forms. Trans fats have been solidly linked to an increased risk of heart disease, so keep these out of your diet at any cost.

Meats:

- ☒ Processed meat: Hold your horses, I know your farmer friend "processes" chickens and makes salami, but that's not we're referring to. We're talking about things like chicken nuggets, frozen pre-prepared meats, anything you get from a fast food establishment, and mass-produced hotdogs, jerky, and cold cuts. There's been a solid link between processed food and colon cancer from the preservation agents. There's also the reality that most of it is full of trans fat and unsavory additives. In small amounts, more traditionally prepared cured meats, like pancetta, nitrate-free bacon, serrano ham, and the like aren't dangerous, but they should be part of a larger diet and not the main source of protein.

- ☒ Breaded meat: Yes, I'm aware that the mob will come at me with pitchforks and torches for this one, but it's true. Breaded meat is delicious - cutlets, fried chicken, schnitzel, and while it is usually deep fat fried, the breading on it is plain unnecessary and bad for a ketogenic diet.

Starches

There's virtually no point in breaking down why you shouldn't have starch on this diet, it should be obvious to you, and if it's not one or both of us needs to reassess our life choices because either you can't read or I can't write or both. Pasta, bread, rice, beans, quinoa, sweet and regular potatoes are all carbohydrate-rich and forbidden. There are times when eating them is acceptable - athletes following the ketogenic diet could get the athletic rush they need from them, but if you're not doing that particular breed of keto, avoid them.

Fruits

See above and replace "starch" with "fruit." Fruit is high in sugar, and that's how trees tricked us into eating it long, long ago. Fruit can, of course, be part of a healthy diet, but it's better to avoid to stay in keto. There are exceptions - olives and avocados of course, and tomato if you're that breed of pedantic who insists on categorizing it with vegetables. Berries, eaten in controlled amounts, can be okay, but okay is not necessarily enough to recommend them, and it's very easy to go overboard. Because of this, they err closer to the side of "don't eat" than "eat."

Vegetables

Avoid anything starchy. This includes potatoes of all breeds, yuca/cassava, breadfruit, corn, squashes. When in doubt, consult nutritional information. Other than that, all non-starchy vegetables have two thumbs up for keto.

Sugars, sweeteners, desserts, etc.

Another no-brainer. Avoid sugar, honey, maple syrup, and artificial sweeteners. Artificial sweeteners have conflicting data - some have displayed insulin spikes, others don't. In my mind, it's better to avoid all of them to avoid the risk altogether. And as tempting as it may to shove a cannoli down your throat the first week, these sugary desserts are also to be avoided like the plague.

Snacks

Things like cheese puffs, potato chips, and candy should all be avoided. Most snacks are made from cheap carbohydrates, and the ones that are meat-based are often more or less suspicious. Stay vigilant when selecting things like store-bought vegetable chips as well.

Drinks:

Soda, sweet tea or coffee, sports drinks, milkshakes are immediately on the chopping block. They're all, by necessity, full of carbohydrates. If you're a fan of kvass, a malted drink from eastern Europe, that is basically unfermented beer and made from bread, so that's to be avoided. Alcoholic beverages in most forms are included too, cocktails are elaborate dressings of liquor and sugar, wine is rotten grape juice, and beer is what happens when you leave your grain harvest bubbling in a metal tank for too long, so those are all out as well.

Conclusion

When this book was written, one of the goals was to be the single, most condensed, easy and fun to read book on the keto diet, covering everything from the very basics, to the science, to how to manage your lifestyle and activity with it, and what to eat while on it. You can go to hundreds of different papers and hundreds of articles to find the precise lifestyle information and scientific knowledge that you need, but hopefully, after compartmentalizing this, you won't have to.

The other goal of this book was to instill a sense of independence into the reader - to give a thorough and sufficient explanation in simple language. Additionally, its aim was to answer any further questions you might have based off the reasoning and explanations you gained from devouring (not literally, good source of fiber though) this book. An old expression says "give a man a fish, he's fed for a day. Teach a man to fish, and he's fed for a lifetime."

It's obvious that keto isn't for everyone - there's more than one way to do it, and it's, by nature, very restrictive. It requires patience, testing, and the ability to suffer through a few weeks of the flu-but-not-the-flu, but if you stick through it, it will come with rewards. Maybe you were trying to wrestle better control over a chronic disease, maybe you were interested in a fast-track way of changing your body composition, of shedding excess weight without having to do hours of grueling cardio and keeping your maxes in the gym, or maybe you were simply trying it out to see what the fuss is about. Whatever reasons you had when picking up this book, I hope that you found what you were looking for.

Finally, if you found this book useful in any way, a review on Amazon is always appreciated!

Intermittent Fasting Mastery

Live a Healthy Life by Following This Complete Guide that Many Men and Women Have Followed, for Transforming Their Lives with the Power of Fasting and the Ketogenic Diet!

By Georgia Bolton

Table of Contents

1. Too much protein at once can kick me out of ketosis

2. You can go keto one day and go off it the next

3. Ketosis is free reign to stuff your craw with deep-fried butter and pork belly

4. Nutrient proportions are set in stone

5. Ketosis is a risk factor for ketoacidosis

6. Ketosis is the ultimate, final way to lose weight

7. Ketosis is a high protein diet

8. Ketosis destroys your heart and valves

9. Keto can cause flu-like symptoms

10. Ketosis exacerbates fatty liver

11. Ketosis carries out a systematic extermination of your gut flora

12. Any fat is good fat

And so it is written

Chapter 11: Good Foods

Fats and oils

Meat, poultry, and seafood

Nuts, Seeds, Legumes, etc.:

Fruits:

Vegetables:

Dairy

Snacks:

Drinks:

Foods to avoid, or at least eat in moderation:

Fats:

Meats:

Starches

Fruits

Vegetables

Sugars, sweeteners, desserts, etc.

Snacks

Drinks:

Introduction

Congratulations on downloading this book and thank you for doing so. This book will help you in understanding the fascinating concept of intermittent fasting and the health benefits it can bring into your life.

Intermittent fasting is a simple concept of managing fasting and eating hours within a day. However, this simple concept can bring amazing changes in your life. This book will explain all the benefits of following intermittent fasting routine and the ways to do so.

This concept has gained great fame for its ability to help in fat burning and weight loss. But, the health benefits of this method are far beyond the small scope of weight loss. It is a way to gain holistic health.

This book will cover the various intermittent fasting protocols in great detail and would also explain other health benefits of following them.

This is a comprehensive guide on intermittent fasting which will tell you each and every aspect of intermittent fasting that you need to know.

You will not only get to know the ways to follow intermittent fasting for successful weight loss and other health benefits but also tell you the things to avoid.

It will tell you the best eating pattern to have while practicing intermittent fasting, the diet that helps in fat burning most and the foods to eat for best results.

You will get to know the different fasting schedules for men and women and the reasons why they should be different.

From best practices to follow during your fast to the right nutrient mix, everything has been given the due weight in this book for making things clear to you.

The safety of practitioners while following intermittent fasting has been given special attention. You will get to know the precautions to take while following intermittent fasting and the things to avoid during your fasts.

You will also get to know the side-effects and the ways you can know if you are heading in the wrong direction.

You will be able to understand the common misconceptions regarding intermittent fasting and why they do not stand the test of reasoning.

To sum it up, this book is your comprehensive guide to understand the power of intermittent fasting and the ways in which it can bring a positive change in your life.

There are plenty of books on this subject on the market, so thanks again for choosing this one! Every effort was made to ensure it is full of as much useful information as possible. Please enjoy!

Chapter 1: Intermittent Fasting—Plain and Simple

It is easy for successful ideas to become an enigma. People start feeling that if something is working and producing amazing results, there must be a great mystery behind that. It has happened with the concept of Intermittent Fasting.

Intermittent Fasting has emerged as a craze in the past few years. It is one of the most effective ways to manage or bring down weight. It can not only help in reducing weight, but it is also very effective in bringing down the belly fat. This charismatic ability of intermittent fasting is earning it a great fan following.

Intermittent Fasting Isn't a New Discovery

It is important to get this fact out of the way at the outset. Intermittent fasting may have resurfaced in the public domain recently, but it is not a new concept discovered by some weight loss guru recently. The basic concept of intermittent fasting has been the way of life for our ancestors for the better part of humanities existence. Yes, you read it right. It has been the existential way of living for our ancestors for thousands of years.

Our ancestors started as hunter-gatherers where they were always on the move. The food availability was scanty, and hence they regularly faced the periods of feasts and famines. That was a time when neither the food storage facilities were available nor there was any knowledge to do so. Therefore, even if they managed to hunt something big, they couldn't store it for long. The natural process of decay and decomposition rendered the food unusable. They had to start fresh most of the time.

It was also the time when they had little advantage over the animals. It is an established fact that we are neither very fast nor very strong. We can't see in the dark as most animals can. We also don't have long claws or teeth. All these things made us inferior. Therefore, hunting is a skill we perfected over a very long period of time. But, before we got skilled in the art of hunting, the availability of food was largely dependent on chance and weakness of the prey.

All this meant is that our ancestors had to go without food for long periods. Whenever they got food, they had to eat as much as they could in one go. The human body has got adapted to this process, and it works very efficiently in this feast and famine cycle. This is the whole concept of intermittent fasting.

Intermittent fasting means that you will get an eating window in which you can eat a reasonable amount of food. Then, there would be a fasting window in which your body will have to go without food. However, during the fasting window, our body starts to function more efficiently as it is very important for survival.

The modern intermittent fasting concept is a refined way of following that cycle of feasting and fasting for better health and functionality. A lot of health issues including the problem of obesity can be resolved by following intermittent fasting.

Origin of Most of the Modern Health Issues

Most of the health issues faced to a very great extent these days have become very severe in the past few decades. Unhealthy lifestyle and poor eating habits are to be blamed for these problems to a very great extent. We have unknowingly turned the boon of food abundance into a bane and that is the main reason behind most of the problems.

The mid-20th century witnessed a great boost in industrialization. We started producing things on a very large scale. Food security improved considerably at least in the developed world. People had more resources, higher financial resources, and the easy availability of food. Bringing food to the table became easier and we overexploited this luxury. We gave in to the pleasures of food, and this has led to most of the problems that trouble us today. There is no control in the amount of food we eat and the number of times we eat it in a day. The physical activity has gone down, and consumption of calories has increased, and this imbalance has led to most of the health issues.

This is a very simplistic explanation of the issue as several health issues also contribute to the problem, but it is important to understand that unregulated eating pattern is at the base of most of the troubles. In this book, we will be discussing all those issues and the ways in which they can be resolved.

Intermittent fasting can help you in resolving these issues as it addresses the core problems and things start to fall in place on their own. If you are troubled with health problems like obesity, diabetes, high blood pressure, and heart ailments, intermittent fasting is the one-stop solution for treating or managing most of the troubles.

The Things That Make Intermittent Fasting Such an Effective Way to Improve Health

Modern medicine has developed by leaps and bounds in the past century. It has found ways to treat some of the most complex health issues. It is working towards finding the cure for deadliest issues like AIDS, Cancer, Cardiovascular damage, and other such problems. However, it is still unable to find a cure for common health disorders like diabetes, high blood pressure, and obesity. There are ways in which you can manage diabetes, blood pressure, and obesity; however, it still doesn't focus on curing these problems completely. The main reason behind this failure is that modern medicine is always busy in treating and suppressing the symptoms. It seems treating these problems completely isn't very profitable for the healthcare industry in the long run.

The doctors explain excellent strategies to manage problems like diabetes, high blood pressure, and obesity and give medicines to keep them under check. However, they fail to explain the strategies to treat these problems completely. All these issues mainly arise when we make compromises with our eating habits and lifestyle. We are reluctant to change our ways, and these problems keep on getting serious. Medicines can help in keeping the symptoms of these diseases low, but they can't change your lifestyle and eating habits and that's why these problems keep on increasing with time.

Intermittent fasting, on the other hand, helps you in bringing a positive change in your eating habits and lifestyle. This has a very profound effect on the things that cause the problems and hence, treating the issues becomes easier.

This book will cover most of these health issues, and the impact intermittent fasting can have on these problems. It will explain the ways in which you can overcome these problems and have a very healthy and fit body that will be able to fight most of these problems on its own.

What Intermittent Fasting Is and What It Isn't

To begin with, intermittent fasting isn't a diet. It is a lifestyle change that can help you in treating the underlying causes of most of the health issues. It is a very subtle, easy, and effective way to address the functional issues your body is facing. It doesn't require calorie counting, reducing the amount of food you eat or starving yourself. It also doesn't ask you to make time taking preparations or spending large sums in taking meticulous classes. It is a simple way of returning to the roots as far as your eating patterns are concerned. Bringing a change in the way you eat, number times you can eat, and the periods in which you can eat is what constitutes intermittent fasting routine. Most importantly, intermittent fasting is a routine and lifestyle change. If you are ready to make some small change in your eating patterns, most of your health issues can be resolved or brought under control, and the way to do so is intermittent fasting.

The Reason for Ineffectiveness of Other Popular Weight Control Measures

Over the course of the past few decades, diets and calorie restrictive regimes have become quite popular. They boast of their amazing abilities to lower the weight and their impact on other health issues. However, the stats tell otherwise. Most people practicing any kind of diet have experienced that diets become ineffective after some time. They need to go on tougher plans, and it becomes impractical. Around 80% of the people who have been on a diet at one point gained more weight than they had originally lost once they got off the diet plan.

There had been several other measures in practice to lose weight. A significant rise in the obesity graph has also led to growing concern in people about its deadliness. In fact, the Centers for Disease Control and Prevention (CDC) report states that out of 900,000 preventable deaths reported annually in the US have around 400,000 cases which could have been prevented if weight could have been lowered. Obesity isn't simply a cosmetic problem as most people think; it brings with itself a number of problems which can become fatal. So, if one manages the weight properly, chances are that untimely death can be averted to a great extent.

This knowledge has caused great concern about managing obesity effectively and thus have surfaced various ways to control it. From gyms to pills and surgeries, people are ready to try almost everything. However, most of these things have largely proven ineffective in reducing obesity pandemic. Global obesity stats show that in spite of so many weight loss measures in practice, the number of people falling in the obese category has tripled in the past four decades. The weight loss industry, on the other hand, has gained a market value of $68 billion in the US alone in this period. If you include the market worth of the European weight loss industry too, the figures reach around $127 billion.

The reason behind the steep rise in the obesity rates despite so much expenditure lies in the fact that most of the popular weight loss methods are difficult to follow in the long run; they require constant work and devotion of time and money. Something or the other is always missing, and hence people fail in keeping their increasing weight in check.

The thing that makes intermittent fasting so effective is the fact that it is easy to follow. Treats the root cause of the problem. Can be practiced without devoting extra time, money, and attention.

Impact of Intermittent Fasting on Your Weight and Overall Health

One very important thing to understand is that you must not consider intermittent fasting as merely a tool to reduce weight. Weight loss is a by-product of improved health which comes naturally. Intermittent fasting is a holistic way to treat most of the health issues causing trouble in your body. Unhealthy lifestyle and poor eating habits cause havoc in your body. They impair your body function and slowly start to interfere with various crucial functions. These ultimately lead to weight gain and other health issues.

Did you know that you can improve your chances of remaining healthy and physically fit simply by increasing insulin sensitivity in your body? Poor eating habits lead to a serious problem called insulin resistance which ultimately leads to diabetes. The main reason for this problem is frequent eating. It means that if you control the frequency of your meals, you can prevent this major trouble. Once your body falls in the trap of insulin resistance, your weight would start increasing uncontrollably. Any number of weight loss efforts would prove to be ineffective if you develop insulin resistance. It will not only cause diabetes and obesity but will also lead to problems like hypertension, high cholesterol, heart problems, chronic inflammation, and other such issues.

Intermittent fasting is one of the most effective ways to prevent insulin resistance. In fact, it can help in converting the negative state of insulin resistance to positive state of insulin sensitivity. If you have higher insulin sensitivity, your body will automatically work towards fighting weight problems and help you in remaining healthy.

Intermittent fasting is also very helpful in improving your body's ability to fight diseases. It helps your digestive system. It improves your cognitive function and you start gaining more muscles while your body loses fat. It means that you will not only get slimmer but also stronger.

Intermittent Fasting Types—Different Paths to Reach Good Health

One of the best things about intermittent fasting is that it allows you to choose the way you want to follow it. It isn't rigid in practice. If you feel that you want to start slow, you can choose an easy intermittent fasting style that will help you in losing weight. Once you get comfortable with the fasting schedules, you can choose longer fasting routines for better and faster results.

All types of intermittent fasting routines have one thing in common and that's their ability to address the inherent problems that lead to poor health. It doesn't matter if you run on a very tight schedule and can't find time to prepare labor intensive diets or sweat for hours in the gym. Intermittent fasting allows you the flexibility to improve your health and lose weight by simply following healthy fasting and eating schedule. If you find it difficult to resist the temptation to eat a few things, you can still lose weight by following intermittent fasting. It doesn't put severe restrictions on the things you can eat and can't eat.

If you can only fast for 2-3 days in a week and that too only for a few hours, you can follow the easier intermittent fasting schedules. If you want to build muscles, intermittent fasting schedules can help you in reducing the body fat faster and gaining muscles.

It means you can choose a suitable intermittent fasting routine as per your convenience and ability to attain the goal of good health. There are several ways to choose from and every way has its specific advantages.

Types of Intermittent Fasting Routines or Protocols

1. **The Leangains Method—16:8 Intermittent Fasting Protocol**

   This is one of the most popular intermittent fasting protocols, and it gets its name due to its ability to help you gain muscle mass while you keep losing the body fat. It is easy and very sustainable in practice. Your body can easily get adjusted this schedule and follow it on a long-term basis without much trouble.

2. **The Warrior Fasting—20:4 Fasting Protocol**

As the name suggests, this intermittent fasting protocol is suitable for the big boys and girls. It is one of the most popular fasting routines within the bodybuilding community and people involved in performance sports. It is very effective in enhancing the production of adrenaline and growth hormones in your body that improve your strength and stamina. It also helps in bulking muscles and lowering the fat in the body.

3. **Eat-Stop-Eat Method**

It is an effective way to lose weight and reduce the risk of several lifestyle disorders without severely changing your lifestyle. If you strongly believe in the advantages of reducing your overall calorie intake but can't follow diets or practice intermittent fasting on a regular basis, this can be one of the best intermittent fasting plans for you. You can fast for any two non-consecutive days of the week and eat in a healthy manner for the rest of the week. The results shown by this method have been very promising.

4. **Alternate Day Fasting—24-Hour Fasting Protocol**

You can consider this fasting protocol as the regular version of the eat-stop-eat method. It requires fasting for the complete 24 hours and then eating normally for the next 24-hours and then resuming the fasts for another 24-hours. In simple words, you will be fasting every other day. This fasting protocol is definitely for the tough souls, but the rewards are handsome and plenty.

5. **The Fast Diet—5:2 Diet Protocol**

This is an odd one out when it comes to actual fasting as it doesn't require you to remain in a complete fasted state. This is more of a calorie restricting method for 2 non-consecutive days a week. However, the results of this method have been great, and this has led to the inclusion of this method in the book.

6. **Spontaneous Meal Skipping**

This is also not a real intermittent fasting protocol, and it isn't structured at all. It is a simple way to listen to your body and skip meals whenever you are not feeling very hungry. However, even skipping meals occasionally can have a very positive impact on your health and that's why this method has got a mention in the book.

We will be discussing all these methods and the correct ways to follow them in detail. You will get to know the specific advantages of each method, and reasons these methods are so effective in their areas.

Chapter 2: Studies that Prove the Effectiveness of Intermittent Fasting

Intermittent fasting may be the oldest way of living humanity has ever known, but scientific research on the subject is very new. The science never paid much attention to the fact that people may be falling sick more due to overeating than malnutrition.

However, this ignorance hasn't been widespread. There are several cultures and religions in the world that have feel following various fasting routines since centuries. They have accepted it as a religious practice to ensure that it is followed by everyone and the whole society can lead a healthy life.

Fasting Followed as Religious Practice and Its Scientific Significance

The reasons for fasting have been different in most religions but it has been invariably present in each one of them.

The Ramadan Fast of the Muslims

Muslims all over the globe observe a mandatory fast for a period of one month every year. In this fast, they begin their fast early in the morning and end the fast after sundown. It gives them 14-16 hours of fasting time while they are leading an active life.

Several studies conducted on the Muslims practicing the fast in these months have proven that their insulin and blood sugar levels improved significantly.

Practitioners lost weight in the months of Ramadan.

Their total cholesterol levels and triglyceride levels also decreased. Women also saw a significant increase in the levels of HDL, the good cholesterol.

The immune system improved in the practitioners, and there was no impact on their kidney function and urine component.

Intermittent Fasting Routines of the Jains

Jainism is a religion practiced in India. It has incorporated intermittent fasting as a way of life for its practitioners.

In this religion, all the followers are expected to eat anything only after saying their morning prayers. This puts their breakfast time around 8-9 in the morning.

The Jain community is a pure vegetarian community, and hence they don't eat anything heavy.

This is a pre-dominantly trader community, and their lifestyle is mostly sedentary. They can eat normally during the day. However, their last meal of the day has to be before sundown. It means most people have their dinner before 5-6 in the evening. They can't eat anything after that.

This gives them 15-16 hours of fasting window.

The rules are the same for men and women; however, the children are not expected to follow this routine.

The advantages:

This is a business community which is involved in very little physical work.

Yet, the community has managed to stay healthy for thousands of years now due to their lifestyle.

They have been following the routine for so long now that it isn't an inconvenience for anyone. It has become a lifestyle.

Study Conducted in 2007 for Prevention of Chronic Diseases Through Alternate Day Fasting

This study showed that intermittent fasting had been effective in lowering the blood pressure in animals.

On animals, it was also noted that alternate day fasting had been effective in reducing the impact of cancer on animals.

However, not much research has been conducted on human beings, and hence the conclusions cannot be drawn.

Studies conducted on some human subject suffering from Type-2 diabetes showed variable results.

A Study Conducted in 2013 to Understand the Impact of Fasting on the Reproductive System

This study was conducted on rats, and it showed that rats when put on fast, demonstrated sexual dysfunction. The impact was more prominent on the female rats.

This is a reason women are advised not to fast for long.

However, this study needs to be done further on human subjects too as the time frame to which the rats were subjected could have been very long when extrapolated in terms of human time as per the respective life cycles.

A Study Conducted in 2017 to Understand the Benefits and Effects of Intermittent Fasting

This study demonstrated that the subjects stopped signs of persistent hunger after a few days. The results of weight loss were, however, inconclusive.

The Intermittent fasting has been a very under-researched subject. Science has now started taking more seriously when promising results have started to come. However, it should never be forgotten that it is an age-old, time-tested way of life and has helped humanity sail through the toughest of times.

Chapter 3: Benefits of Intermittent Fasting

Intermittent fasting is a holistic way to treat your body. Its benefits are no way restricted to weight loss. In fact, as I have stated earlier, weight loss is simply a by-product of the good health that you acquire through intermittent fasting.

Intermittent fasting has a profound effect on several health parameters, and it helps in improving the functioning of your body. Your overall health biomarkers would start improving as soon as you begin your fasting. You would start noticing significant changes in the way your body functions and also in your energy levels.

This chapter will explain the changes in various areas in your health and the reasons for those positive changes.

Improved Insulin Sensitivity

Insulin sensitivity is a term that will be used several times in the book, and therefore, it is important that you clearly understand its significance in your health. Insulin is one of the most important hormones in your body. It has some crucial jobs to perform that affect your weight and fat accumulation too.

Insulin is a hormone released by the pancreas. It performs several functions, but two important jobs performed by it can mean life and death for all of us.

Whenever you eat anything, the food is processed by your body, and it is converted into glucose. The glucose is a ready form of energy that your cells can absorb and use immediately without the requirement of any further processing. So, the process is simple, the glucose mixes in your bloodstream and raises the blood glucose levels. The blood travels all over your body, and hence the glucose is made available to each and every cell of the body to utilizing the energy. The mitochondria in your cells can use this glucose for running the cell functions. However, there is a catch. The cells cannot absorb glucose on their own. There is a barrier that stops them. It's like the cells are locked and they need a key to open them for absorbing the glucose. Insulin is that key which allows the absorption of glucose by cells.

So, the first job of insulin is to bind with the cells and allow them to absorb glucose. Without insulin, your cells will be unable to absorb glucose and starve.

The second crucial job of insulin is to bring down high blood sugar levels. Consumption of food increases the release of glucose into your body. This elevates your blood sugar levels. This is a process that gets repeated after every meal. Insulin lowers the blood sugar levels by storing the excess glucose in a form of glycogen and fat in your body as consistently high blood sugar levels for long can be fatal. It is the main fat storage hormone in your body.

If you fear the accumulation of bulging tires around the abdomen or flapping thighs, then also, this is the hormone you should worry about messing around. This is a hormone which isn't good neither when it is abundant nor when it is in short supply.

It is a very important hormone. You stand no chance of healthy survival if there are any problems related to insulin in your body or the insulin levels are off the chart.

However, I digress. Let us go through the energy process once again. Every meal that you consume ultimately releases glucose. It takes your body anywhere around 8-12 hours to utilize the glucose in the bloodstream and normalize the blood sugar levels. As soon as the blood sugar levels go down, the insulin levels also dissipate. The pancreas in your body will keep producing and pumping insulin as long as the blood sugar levels don't get normal.

Problem #1

It begins with the habit of frequent snacking and having late night meals. The thing is that your cells can't accept glucose on their own. They need insulin to unlock them. It acts as a messenger that helps in glucose absorption. However, when you start having meals every few hours, insulin is always present in the blood. The cells get so used to the insulin that they stop responding to it readily. This is called the incremental threat effect of overexposure. It means that if there is a healthy exposure to a thing, the reaction would be positive, this is called the mere exposure effect. However, when the exposure becomes constant, everything starts developing a distaste. They become insensitive.

This is what happens with the cells. When the insulin is always present in the blood, the cells stop showing their receptiveness to bond with the insulin. This means that although the blood sugar levels in your bloodstream are high, and the insulin is also present, the cells don't show great receptiveness to insulin. Hence, your blood sugar level remains high, and your cells also don't get proper glucose. This is an alarming problem. The pancreas senses the high blood sugar level, and it starts pumping more and more insulin. For utilizing the same amount of blood sugar, your body starts needing much more insulin. This problem is called **Insulin Resistance**.

It puts a lot of pressure on your pancreas and also leads to a problem called prediabetes which is a primary stage of diabetes.

Problem #2

Once you develop insulin resistance, the levels of insulin also remain very high in your blood. Insulin is also a fat storage hormone. It means that by the time the insulin levels are high, your body will not start burning body fat in any condition. You may run on the treadmill for hours, but you wouldn't be burning fat. You would at the most exhaust the glucose in the bloodstream but wouldn't be able to metabolize fat. Therefore, burning fat would remain a big problem in the case of insulin resistance.

Problem #3

There are several hormones that can help in fat burning. However, the production of these hormones can only take place once the insulin levels go down. If your body has insulin resistance and you are having frequent meals, that is not going to happen anytime soon.

Problem #4

Because your cells stop responding to insulin readily, the pancreas has to produce more and more insulin. This puts an unnecessary load on the pancreas. It can also lead to the development of pancreatitis.

Problem #5

Consistently, high blood sugar levels can become a cause of great concern. It can cause fatigue, swelling, and several other serious issues including multiple organ failure.

Insulin resistance is a problem that needs to be feared. There can be several reasons behind insulin resistance; however, frequent snacking is a big one among them.

How Intermittent Fasting Helps in Developing Insulin Sensitivity

The biggest contribution of intermittent fasting to your health is that it helps in the development of insulin sensitivity. The main reason behind the development of insulin resistance is its overexposure to the cells. It happens as your body needs to constantly pump insulin to stabilize the blood sugar levels.

Following an Intermittent Fasting routine would involve remaining in a fasted state for a considerably longer duration. Let us consider the 16-hour fasts as they are one of the easiest routines to follow.

Now suppose, you started your day at 7 in the morning.

Had your breakfast around 9 in the morning.

Had your lunch at 1 in the afternoon.

Finished your dinner by 5 in the evening.

This is the time your fasting window would begin.

You finished your 8-hour eating window. Your body takes anywhere between 8-12 hours to stabilize the blood glucose levels. It means that your insulin levels would start getting low after 5-6 hours of your last meal. Between 8-12 hours, the insulin levels would reduce considerably. However, the fasting window is of 16 hours. This means that your body will maintain low insulin levels anywhere between 6-10 hours. This gives your cells time away from constant insulin badgering at their doors. This is the simple, most important thing that would help your cells in developing insulin sensitivity as the problem of overexposure of insulin would end. The next time when you have your meals, the cells would respond better to insulin stimuli.

Therefore, intermittent fasting can help in a big way in the development of **Insulin Sensitivity**.

Faster Fat Burning

Fat burning is a very unique process. Your body can run on two types of fuel viz. glucose and fat. The food that we eat is mainly composed of carbohydrates, protein, and fat. Your body processes the food that you eat and converts it into glucose. Glucose is an easy to burn fuel, and your body loves to stay on it.

The fat stored in your body isn't toxic waste. Your body has passed through a great deal of evolution to learn to store fat. It can use this fat to provide energy when the ready form of energy from glucose is not available. It is a part of the survival mechanism of your body. However, your body will never start burning fat without a cause. It likes to keep it stored for the times when you are really short on energy. Hibernating animals use their body fat to survive for months while they are sleeping in adverse conditions.

However, to make your body use the fat as a form of energy, you will have to starve it for a considerable amount of time and cut-off the ready supply of energy. This is where intermittent fasting comes into play.

Before we move any further, you will have to understand the mechanism of fat burning.

When you are eating frequently, your body keeps getting the ready supply of glucose. It doesn't matter whether you lower the supply of energy or not. Until your body is getting glucose, it would not burn fat. This is where the diets fail to hit the nail.

People have a misconception that if they lower their calorie intake, their bodies will have no other option than to burn fat for energy. Remember, diets and calorie restrictive regimes only reduce the calorie intake; they never completely cut the supply. When your calorie intake gets low, your body senses that there is a problem. If it keeps running on the normal calorie consumption mode, it will be starved of energy. This is where it makes a move and lowers your metabolic rate. It means that it lowers the amount of energy you require to run your body. This is a reason people start feeling lethargic, tired, and energy drained when they are on diets. However, the body doesn't burn the fat as it simply can't. You lower the amount of food you consume in the meals, but you still have a greater number of meals in a day at short intervals. This keeps your insulin levels high. It is a fat storage hormone, and hence till it is present no fat burning would take place.

Following intermittent fasting helps you in cutting off the energy supply completely at least temporarily. However, your body needs energy supplies at regular intervals as cells can only store small amounts of energy. To run the vital functions, your body has no other alternative than to metabolize the fat stores for providing energy and hence the fat burning takes place.

To initiate fat burning, you will need to stop the continuous supply of energy even in small amounts. This is what intermittent fasting does. It imposes a curfew on ready glucose supply.

When you remain in the fasted state for a bit longer, your body also starts the production of some fat burning hormones. Hormones like the Human Growth Hormone (hGH) and adrenaline are produced that also speed up the fat metabolization. It is important to note here that these hormones cannot be produced by your body till there is insulin present in your bloodstream.

The production of hGH also increases when the levels of "Ghrelin" the hunger hormones are also high. This is also a condition which intermittent fasting fulfills as you remain hungry for long.

Therefore, you can lose weight and burn fat faster by following intermittent fasting protocols.

Impact of Intermittent Fasting on Heart Health

The heart is one of the most vital organs in our body. It pumps blood day in and day out. However, it is a very sensitive organ. Various processes in your body have a very profound impact on the health of your heart. For instance, if your blood pressure remains too high, it will put a lot of pressure on the heart and would cause damage to it. If your blood sugar levels remain consistently high, they will lead to stiffening of muscles and that would also lead to heart injuries. From chronic inflammation in your body to chronic stress, all these things cause injuries to the heart and the vessels carrying blood to the heart.

TV advertisements, product sales scripts, and even medical science have led us to believe that cholesterol deposits in the heart vessels lead to heart issues.

Cholesterol blocks the blood carrying vessels and that causes most of the problems. Therefore, you must lower your consumption of fat and cholesterol. The whole concept is misleading, and they are telling only one part of the story.

It is correct that most of the heart problems are caused due to blockage of the heart vessels by cholesterol. However, cholesterol is not the kind of villain it is projected to be. In fact, it is very important for the proper functioning of your body.

Did you know that it is the material from which most of the cells are made?

Did you also know that most of the important hormones are made from cholesterol?

Did you know that cholesterol is the repairing material for your heart?

Whenever your heart vessels get damaged due to high blood pressure, chronic stress or any other kind of injury, cholesterol rushes to repair the damage. It gets deposited on the artery walls as plaque. When the damage is frequent, the plaque deposit gets thicker and leads to heart attacks. However, it was never the primary reason for heart problems in the first place.

Another common misconception is that by removing the fat and cholesterol from your food you can prevent heart damage. It is not entirely true.

Dietary cholesterol plays a very insignificant role in causing heart damage. It is simply used for providing energy. Most of the damage is caused by the LDL, VLDL, and triglycerides which are bad cholesterols. Their production is high when the levels of antioxidants go very low in your body, and your body has very high levels of blood sugar.

Intermittent fasting helps your body in improving the overall health biomarkers that lead to heart injuries. It plays an important role in lowering the levels of LDL, VLDL, and triglycerides as they are used by your body to produce energy when the glucose supply is low.

You can give a great boost to your heart health by doing regular exercise as it helps in making the vessels carrying blood to your heart more flexible.

A healthy lifestyle with low stress also helps in reducing the injuries to the heart.

Some of the Important Roles That Intermittent Fasting Plays in Ensuring Improved Heart Health Are:

Promotes Insulin Sensitivity

Insulin resistance is among the leading reasons for common heart injuries and blockage. When your insulin levels remain high very consistently, it directs a lot of harmful lipids to your heart walls that lead to blockage. Insulin resistance also leads to chronic inflammations and that produces cytokines which add to the problem. It is also responsible for high blood pressure which is a major cause of heart damage.

Intermittent fasting is very effective in reversing insulin resistance and that helps in controlling the problems that cause heart damage.

Helps in Controlling High Blood Pressure

High blood pressure is like the cat which is very difficult to tame. It can occur due to a number of reasons. However, one big reason for high blood pressure is insulin resistance. Once your insulin levels are under control, it gets easier for you to manage your blood pressure. The more you have control over your blood pressure, the lower will be the damage to your heart. High blood pressure can also occur due to problems like water retention in the body. Intermittent fasting can also help you in taking care of this issue as well.

Better Stress Resistance

Stress also plays an important role in causing damage to the heart. Intermittent fasting plays a very important role in lowering the risk of damage from stress. When you do any kind of fasting, you expose your body to lower levels of stress. This stress acts as positive stress, and it enables your heart in absorbing stress at low levels. Therefore, when blood pressure, insulin resistance, and other such things cause stress, your heart is better equipped to handle it and doesn't show a shock reaction. Hence, sudden damage due to stress is low.

Reduces the Amount of Free Fatty Acids

Free fatty acids also cause the highest amount of blockage in the arteries. The free fatty acids are released by the visceral fat stored in your body. The higher the amount of visceral fat, the greater would be the amount of free fatty acids. They can cause great damage. However, free fatty acids are not produced without reason. Your body can use them for producing energy under the right circumstances, and intermittent fasting helps in the creation of such circumstances.

Intermittent fasting creates short energy demands in your body. When there is no other source of energy, your body can use these free fatty acids for producing energy, and hence the risk from them will reduce. On the contrary, you will be able to benefit from them.

The Boost in the Production of Human Growth Hormone (hGH)

The Human Growth Hormone (hGH) is one hormone that can make a huge difference in your weight loss efforts. It is a hormone that your body produces to achieve several growth goals.

The production of growth hormone is very high in kids as they are growing. It reaches its peak when they reach teenage as their bodies start growing very fast. However, once a person crosses the teenage, the rate of production of growth hormone gets low as one isn't growing anymore and only aging.

It is a hormone that plays a very crucial role in burning fat, brings anti-aging effects, and healing injuries. These are the reasons that the production of this hormone never stops completely; it simply gets low. Your body produces the growth hormone in short bursts.

The production is very high in the following conditions:

1. When the insulin levels in your blood are very low
2. When you are sleeping and hungry
3. When you do high-intensity exercise
4. When you face any injury or trauma

The fourth condition is not applicable as you wouldn't want to increase your hGH levels at the cost of an injury. However, the other three conditions get fulfilled when you follow intermittent fasting.

Intermittent fasting leads to the development of better insulin sensitivity, and hence your blood glucose levels stabilize faster. This would mean that the insulin levels also start getting low at a better rate. The fasting also ensures that you remain empty stomach for longer, and this also facilitates the production of hGH. In the last legs of your fasting, you are mostly asleep, and hence the hGH production increases. If you couple that with some high-intensity exercise, your body will be able to produce hGH in high quantities.

This hormone can burn fat faster than anything else. It specifically helps in burning fat and building muscles. A study conducted by the American College of Cardiology shows that intermittent fasting can lead to an increase in production of hGH up to 2000% in men and 1400% in women.

Some advantages of high hGH levels are:
- ✓ Faster burning of the abdominal fat tissues
- ✓ Better muscle buildup
- ✓ Increase in stamina during high-intensity interval training
- ✓ Better immune system
- ✓ Better mood regulation
- ✓ Strong anti-aging effects
- ✓ Faster healing of injuries
- ✓ Increase in libido
- ✓ Higher production of anabolic hormones

Therefore, you can burn the belly fat faster if your hGH levels are high.

Better Satiety Through Improved Leptin Sensitivity

Have you ever wondered why people who are obese tend to have a higher appetite? This is beyond reason as these are the people who should eat the least as their energy demands are low. Yet, they find it difficult to resist food when it is in front and that keeps adding on weight to them.

If you have been laughing at them or pitying them, then you are wrong. It is something beyond their control. All this happens when one hormone gets out of control and starts messing with the brain.

The fat cells in the body release a hormone called "Leptin." This is the satiety hormone, and its main job is to instruct the brain to stop eating as the fat stores are high. The higher the fat content in the body, the greater would be the release of leptin hormone, and you should start feeling full faster. However, this is where the problem begins.

When a person has too much fat, the release of leptin is also very high. The problem starts when there is inflammation in the fat cells. This causes the fat cells to keep releasing the leptin hormone at moderate levels all the time. This means that your brain is constantly getting the message to stop eating as the fat stores are abundant. The problem of overexposure starts creating a problem here too.

When the release of leptin is constant, your brain stops registering its signal.

The levels of leptin should be the lowest when you are hungry and highest when you are full. The inflammation in the fat cells leads to the moderate release of leptin all the time, and hence brain is unable to distinguish the signal. This is a state called leptin resistance. That is why obese people never feel satisfied. They can eat immediately after eating something.

There are three factors that cause leptin resistance:

1. **Consistent Release of Leptin Hormone:** If your fat cells remain consistently high, your brain would stop registering them, and it would lead to leptin resistance.

2. **Inflammation in the Fat Cells:** If there is inflammation in the fat cells, they would keep releasing leptin, and it would also cause leptin resistance.

3. **High Amount of Free Fatty Acids:** High-fat deposits in the body release more free fatty acids. They can interfere with the ability of the brain to recognize the leptin hormone and that would also lead to leptin resistance.

There are 2 main ways in which Intermittent Fasting helps:

It Stops Chronic Inflammation: Intermittent fasting plays a crucial role in fighting inflammation in your body. It helps in bringing down the free fatty acids which are the main culprits behind inflammation. The lower the inflammation, the greater will be leptin sensitivity. Bringing down free fatty acids also helps in the cause as they stop misleading the brain.

Lowers the Release of Leptin Through Extended Fasting Hours: When you fast for longer hours, your leptin levels go down automatically as the constant release is sparked by frequent eating. When your brain doesn't have to bear the constant knocking of the hormone, it gets better at recognizing it.

The more sensitive your brain is to leptin, the lower will be your urge to eat anything. This will help you in fasting as well as managing weight.

Taming of the Hunger Hormone "Ghrelin"

The villain of this story is "Sugar." I started the topic with an unusual thing. The reason is that the ghrelin hormone is supposed to be the good hormone. It performs several crucial functions like makes you feel hungry when your stomach is empty. It also boosts the production of growth hormone. High ghrelin levels can also boost your cognitive function. Your body would be able to regulate insulin better, and your heart would also function better if your ghrelin release is normal. However, that doesn't happen, and the reason is sugar.

The ghrelin is your hunger hormone. When your stomach is empty, the levels of ghrelin are the highest. As you keep eating your ghrelin levels go down, and you stop feeling hungry anymore. The release of ghrelin and leptin is inversely proportional. When the ghrelin levels are high, your leptin levels should be low. When your leptin levels go high, the ghrelin levels must go down as you would start feeling satiety by them. However, that also doesn't happen and that is also due to sugar.

When you feel hungry and your gut starts producing ghrelin you eat. However, if your food of choice is any kind of sugar-laced product, you would be getting empty calories that would raise your blood sugar levels but wouldn't give your gut anything substantial to process, and hence it would keep releasing ghrelin.

The leptin levels remain consistently moderate if you keep eating sweets as they are a reason for inflammation. So, even after eating a lot, your leptin levels would never rise too high. The gut would not get a message to lower the ghrelin levels. You would overeat and load too many empty calories that would also cause obesity.

Consistently, high levels of ghrelin would slowly start decreasing the impact of the hormone and all other functions would get affected.

Intermittent fasting helps you in putting a stop although temporary to consistent loading of sugar into your system. The longer you remain away from sugar, the better your ghrelin release would be. Remember, this hormone affects the functioning of several other hormones and functions and messing with it can be dangerous.

Reduction in Chronic Inflammation

Chronic inflammation is dangerous. It can lead to problems like heart diseases, hypertension, thyroid issues, obesity, chronic pain, diabetes, migraines, and even cancers. Not only this, problems like autoimmune diseases like ulcerative colitis, rheumatoid arthritis, multiple sclerosis, and Crohn's disease are also caused by chronic inflammation.

High amounts of oxidative stress, free fatty acids, triglycerides, LDL, and VLDL in your blood lead to chronic inflammation.

The risk of chronic inflammation increases if:

- You are overweight
- You eat unhealthy things
- You are leading a stressful life
- You have a sedentary lifestyle

Intermittent fasting can help you in managing the oxidating stress and free fatty acids. It also helps your body in using up triglycerides, LDL, and VLDL in your blood for producing energy. This lowers the risk of chronic inflammations, and you can avoid these problems.

Intermittent fasting is a healthy way of living, and it also helps in reducing your weight which in itself is a reason for inflammations. Better lifestyle also lowers the risk.

Help in Diabetes

In general, all the diseases are bad. They limit your capabilities and take the fun out of life. You lose time, money, and health. However, those diseases are especially bad for which there is no permanent cure. They simply stick to you. They become lifelong disorders, and diabetes is one among such problems.

Serious and poor management of diabetes can have serious implications. We all know that high blood sugar levels are bad, and they can even cause multiple organ failures and death. But low blood sugar is not any less dangerous. It can cause seizures, coma, or even death. Therefore, proper management of diabetes is crucial.

The problem with diabetes is that it simply sticks with the patients for the whole life. It means that the patient becomes dependent on medications and insulin injections. Conventional medicine has no other way to treat this problem.

Intermittent fasting can be a savior for people suffering from diabetes or prediabetes. The US alone has more than 110 million people with diabetes or prediabetes.

It isn't without fact that intermittent fasting can help in lowering the impact of diabetes or reversing it. To make it clearer, it is important to understand the underlying causes of diabetes and the ways intermittent fasting helps in them.

Helps in Maintaining Healthy Blood Sugar Levels

High blood sugar is the main problem in diabetes. Your body cannot bear high levels of blood sugar. It causes microhemorrhage in the eyes, kidney, and heart vessels. This means that the vessels in these organs start to leak blood. To counter that, a special type of protein material called fibrinogen increases in your blood that leads to clotting. However, excessive clotting of blood can cause obstructions in the vessels carrying blood to heart, kidney, and eyes. Strokes, high blood pressure, impaired vision, and hardening of the arteries are some of the immediate effects. It ultimately leads to organ failure if blood sugar levels do not come down. High blood sugar also leads to fatty liver and may also cause liver cirrhosis.

Intermittent fasting helps in this area a lot as it reduces the risk of frequent blood sugar spikes. Your blood sugar rises every time you eat food. It is the result of glucose from the food mixing in your bloodstream. Intermittent fasting limits your eating windows, and this lowers the risk of frequent blood sugar spikes. Additionally, following a high-fat low-carb diet is also important. It helps your body in running on fat fuel rather than glucose provided by carbohydrates.

Helps in Decreasing Insulin Resistance

Insulin is the main hormone that regulates your blood sugar and puts it to good use. As soon as your blood sugar increases, the pancreas starts off-loading insulin to help in the absorption of that blood sugar. The real problem begins when the cells stop responding to insulin. This is a problem that can happen due to overexposure of insulin, and it is called insulin resistance. In that case, the pancreas needs to pump more and more insulin even for absorbing small amounts of blood sugar. Additional insulin shots may also be required to fulfill the need for insulin. The solution to this problem is that your body needs to become more sensitive to insulin. However, our eating habits act against developing insulin sensitivity. People wrongly believe that if they stop eating sugar, their blood sugar levels would go down. This is not going to happen. Either you eat sugar or not, if you are eating, your body will convert it into sugar, and your pancreas will keep pumping insulin to process it.

This is where intermittent fasting can come to the rescue. It helps in bringing prolonged fasting hours where food intake completely stops. Your blood sugar levels go down in 8-12 hours and so do your insulin needs. Around 16 hours of fasting creates a gap of 4-8 hours when your bloodstream was free of excess insulin. It helps in the redeveloping of insulin sensitivity. Your body starts responding better to the insulin produced by the pancreas and doesn't need extra insulin to be injected.

Gives a Chance to the Pancreas to Recover

Excessive production of insulin puts the pancreas under a lot of stress. The pancreas has very important functions. It produces insulin, glucagon, and various enzymes. Extra burden on pancreas can lead to several complications. Pancreatic insufficiency is one among them. This will lower the ability of the pancreas to produce insulin, glucagon, and enzymes.

Intermittent fasting helps by giving your pancreas the time to recover. The time when you are not eating during intermittent fasting, your pancreas does not need to pump more insulin. After a certain amount of time, your body needs to burn fat and for that, the pancreas produces glucagon. This changes the function. Created insulin sensitivity and pancreas can also recover.

Helps in Weight Loss

It is an open secret that weight loss is among the most effective ways to successfully manage diabetes. Intermittent fasting leads to weight loss in a number of ways and, therefore, gives you much-needed respite from the harmful effects of diabetes.

Promotes Anti-aging

We all want to stay young forever. We know that's an unreasonable demand, but something simply snatches away our youth much earlier than it should go, and I believe there is nothing more unreasonable than that. People consider early aging only to be a cosmetic issue, but it isn't. Aging is much more of a physiological problem too. Aging occurs when the damage to your body is higher than the normal rate at which it can regenerate things. The regeneration process slows down as we grow, but it has accelerated at an early age then you are looking for the problem at wrong places.

Three most important reasons for faster aging are:
- High free radical damage
- Oxidative stress
- Low Glycosaminoglycans (GAG) levels

You already know that intermittent fasting can help you in reducing the free radical damage and oxidative stress. The GAG is a chemical that is responsible for keeping the collagen of your skin hydrated. Once the levels of GAG go down, your skin starts to wrinkle and sag. This GAG production is controlled by another hormone produced in your liver by the name of IGF-1. Intermittent fasting is the only known way to boost the production of this hormone.

Autophagy

Autophagy is a new term that has come in the limelight as a Japanese scientist by the name of Yoshinori Oshumi recently published his research on this matter in 2016 and won a Nobel prize for it. This concept states that your body has an innate ability to treat most of its problems on its own. The only thing required is the right conditioning.

Our lifestyle these days has become such that we are providing everything to our body in excess. This has made our bodies inefficient in its functioning as it doesn't need rationing. However, our body has the ability to run more efficiently if it is forced to do so.

He states that in case our body senses a shortage of supply of energy, the first thing it does is that it starts optimizing all the processes. It is important for running the body longer on less energy. This process of optimization of the processes is called autophagy.

The beauty of this process lies in the fact that it doesn't waste anything and starts using every part of your cell to regenerate new cells. It even starts purging all the pathogens, germs, harmful bacteria, and fungi in your body as they are also using up energy. Most of the problems start getting resolved in the process.

It means even the toughest physiological problems and chronic inflammations will get treated on their own if your body starts the process of autophagy.

The requirement for autophagy is that you must temporarily cut the energy supply of your body from outside. It means you must stop eating. When you eat, you are not only feeding your body, you are also feeding all the pathogens, infections, chronic inflammations, cancer cells, and other malice.

Intermittent fasting can help you in starting the process of autophagy. It gives your body the required break it needs and that's why intermittent fasting is so effective in treating most of the problems.

Some people believe that actual autophagy only starts when you fast for long. However, studies have shown that autophagy can also begin when you fast for shorter durations like 12-16 hours.

This process can take you toward good health and intermittent fasting can be the way to achieve it.

Chapter 4: Intermittent Fasting Protocols

As we had discussed earlier, intermittent fasting is simply a pattern of fasting and feasting. The health benefits would largely depend upon the number of hours you fast, the kind of food you eat, and the lifestyle you follow.

Intermittent fasting in itself is a complete method. It means that if weight loss is a goal, you will achieve it irrespective of the fact that you exercise, or you don't. You will lose belly fat even if you are not able to ditch the fast food completely. However, these are the factors which have a significant impact on your weight loss speed. Therefore, if you are following a healthy lifestyle, doing a bit of exercise and eating healthy, your weight loss journey would be a lot smoother and faster. You will also be able to remain healthy and fit for longer with very little extra effort.

Weight loss is a very small part of the advantages that intermittent fasting has to offer. We have discussed all the health benefits that you can get by following intermittent fasting routines, and hence you must keep them in account while comparing intermittent fasting with any other diet plan.

You can keep shorter and easier fasts or go for tougher fasting protocols; the choice would always be yours. However, you must always remember that while you can tax your body, you must not try to challenge it. Our bodies don't like getting shaken to a jolt. The reactions are sometimes intense. From steep hormonal changes to erratic reactions, your body may react in abnormal ways if you will try to take up something to which your body isn't accustomed. Therefore, you must always start with easier intermittent fasting schedules and then move on to the next one when the body gets used to it.

The Preparation—Getting Rid of the Habit of Snacking

If there is one thing that has caused the highest amount of damage to our health in modern times, it is the habit of frequent snacking. Some so-called came up with the idea that frequent snacking habits keep the metabolism running, and the food producing industry started pushing it with its full might as it suited their business. The more frequent the snacking habit is, the better their business would be. It helps the cereal making companies, it helps the companies that produce ready-to-eat products, and it even helps the fast food industry.

The benefits of frequent snacking were pushed so hard through commercials and campaigns that people started treating it as gospel truth. Probably the saying "A lie told often enough becomes a truth" is true after all. However, it is one of the main reasons behind the obesity epidemic plaguing the whole world today.

The habit of frequent snacking is also one of the biggest roadblocks you will face that deters people from fasting or staying hungry. We are actually habitual of a dangerous cocktail. First, we like to eat frequently at very short intervals. Second, most of the times, the essential component of these snacks is refined sugar. These two things lead to cravings for food. It means you will keep on feeling the need to eat even after short food intervals. These needs are called food cravings and initially, they make remaining in the fasted state very tough.

So, to follow intermittent fasting in a proper way, you will have to try to ditch these two things as much as possible. If you can completely leave them well and good, or else, try to maintain a safe distance and don't let them overpower you.

The best way to prepare your body for intermittent fasting is to eliminate the snacks from your schedule completely. It means that you will have to manage with only 3 meals a day and nothing besides that. It looks tough and let us examine the reasons that make it tough.

On any given day, we all have got into a habit of eating 6-8 times a day. For some people, the number of times they eat in a day can be even higher. However, if we consider the number of times that we spike our insulin levels in a day, the instances can go as high as 10-15 times. Before you let this settle in your mind, you must also remember that every time your insulin levels are spiked, your fat burning abilities diminish considerably. Your body becomes more eager to accumulate fat than to burn it. The insulin spike in your body would take place every time you ingest anything that contains calories. It means sipping a cup of tea, coffee, or soda can spike your insulin levels. Not only this, chewing a sweet gum, a candy, popcorn, or anything else containing calories will also have the same effect. Now, considering all these facts, put some pressure on your brain and try to recollect the number of times you caused insulin spike yesterday. If you have reached a higher number than we have discussed, I won't be surprised.

On average, our eating schedules go as follows:

No.	Description	Time
1	Pre-Breakfast snacks	6-8 am
2	Breakfast	8-10 am
3	Morning Snack	10-11 am
4	Lunch	1-2 pm
5	Evening Snack	4-5 pm
6	Dinner	7-10 pm

7	Post-Dinner snacks	9-11 pm

These are the times when we are eating things that are loaded with calories. Our meals are full of refined sugar in various forms that also aggravates the problem. Higher the number of times you eat in a day, the more difficult it will get for you to remain in the fasted state.

The first thing that you must do in order to follow any kind of fasting schedule in any considerable manner is to eliminate all kinds of snacks from your food. There is no getting around this point. If you have a habit of frequent having frequent snacks, you will experience powerful cravings that will be difficult to avoid. You must eliminate the snacks from your routine and stick to 3 meals a day routine. This will help you in fighting with cravings, and your system will be able to get better at treating insulin. If you are not able to stay away from snacks, fasting may get very difficult for you to follow, and food will always remain the main thing at the back of your mind.

The Leangains Method—16:8 Intermittent Fasting Protocol

This is one of the most famous intermittent fasting protocols. As I have already told, this intermittent fasting protocol gets the name Leangains from its ability to help you in losing fat and gaining lean muscle mass. Both of these things have been unheard of in the weight loss industry till now. The methods which caused any amount of fat loss also undoubtedly led to the loss of muscle mass too. The reasons for the same are simple. When you start restricting energy supply to your body, the first thing it tries to use for energy is the most similar looking structure, and protein definitely fits the bill. Carbohydrate is the easiest to break and a favorite fuel of your body. After it, comes protein, and the fat is always the last choice as your body requires a completely different process to burn it.

The Leangains method compels your body to start burning the fat. The fat in your body is a very stable fuel. Burning even a small amount of fat can provide a lot of energy, and it releases the least amount of toxic waste. However, your body can't keep burning carbohydrate and fat at the same time. So, while your body is really burning the fat, there will be no substantial loss of the muscle mass. In fact, if you engage in high-intensity interval training while practicing intermittent fasting, you will be able to build muscles faster as it helps in the production of two important hormones called the growth hormones and the adrenaline. Both these hormones greatly enhance the ability of your body to build muscle and stamina. So effectively, your body would lose the fat accumulated at your belly and thighs and build muscles.

After you have been practicing intermittent fasting for a while, you might notice that you weigh almost the same on the scale although you are feeling you are getting slimmer. If that is the case, there is all the reason for you to be happy as your body would have adapted itself to the fat burning process. It would be burning fat and that would make you get slimmer. However, you also start to gain muscle mass. The muscles are more compact and heavier than fat and that's why although you may look slim you may not weigh less but it is a blessing in disguise and the dream of millions.

The Process

This method is called the 16:8 fasting protocol, and the reason for it is that you will need to remain in the fasted state for 16 hours a day and have an eating window of 8 hours. This schedule is for men who want to follow this protocol. For women, the ideal protocol would be 14:10 with 14-hours of fasting window and 10-hours of eating window. Several studies conducted on women have shown that shorter fasts work better with the hormonal system of the body of a female. So, although this protocol is popularly known as 16:8, it is effectively 14:10 for women and that shouldn't be confused.

The Fasting Window

This is the time people are worried about the most. Although 16 hours of fasting may look like a big number, by managing your eating schedule well, you can pass it very easily.

The most important things about easily passing the fasting window are the timings of beginning the fast. It is always the best to time your fasts as per your morning routines. If you like to wake up early in the morning, then you must try to begin your fasting early in the evening. For instance, if you wake up at 6 in the morning, then your fasting must begin by 6-7 in the evening at the latest. The earlier it begins, the least amount of restraint you will have to apply on your urge to eat something.

The 16:8 Fasting for Morning People

Suppose you begin your fasting at 6 in the evening. If you are a morning person and wake up early, you will have to sleep early. This means you will go to bed by 10-11 at night. This would give you 4-5 hours of gap between dinner and sleeping. This is an undisputed fact that having dinner a few hours before going to bed is the best for your health. Having dinner 4-5 hours before the bedtime makes it highly probable that you will remain in a physically active state. It will also make the digestion process faster and smoother. By the time you will go to bed, food processing in your body would be nearing its completion stage, and it is among one of the best things for your body.

The 4-5 hours before you go to sleep would be easy as you'd feel no real urge to eat during this time. Starting the fasting at 6 would mean that by 7 in the morning you would have passed a majority of the time effortlessly in your sleep. Women would only need to continue their fasting for another hour and for men, there would be 3 more hours to pass before they can break that fast.

Once you start practicing intermittent fasting, you would stop feeling the urge to eat anything specifically in this time as your body gets used to the routine and your gut starts timing the release of 'ghrelin', the hunger hormone, as per your eating schedules. However, if you still feel the hunger pangs, you can have unsweetened black tea, black coffee, green tea, or fresh lime drink without sugar. These beverages would help you in suppressing your hunger without adding calories to your system. These are not only safe beverages but also provide a lot of antioxidants. You must try to continue your fast for as long as possible as the longer you would continue your fasting, the better would be the results.

The last few hours of fasting are crucial for fat burning. This is the time when the production of the hGH and adrenaline is at its peak in your body. These two hormones can help you in burning fat big time. Even a small amount of exercise will lead to terrific results.

I'd highly recommend exercise during this period. If you can do high-intensity interval training, it is the best as it leads to faster fat burning and muscle buildup. However, if you don't have the time or inclination to do that, even simple cardio exercises, aerobics, or yoga would also be very beneficial.

The women can break their fast after 14 hours, and men can do that after 16 hours of fasting.

Your eating window should ideally begin after the given hours of fasting. However, there is no reason to be very rigid about the timing. You can take the liberty of an hour if you feel the hunger to be uncontrollable and try to fast for longer the next day. This is something that would feel tough initially but would become effortless later on.

The Eating Window

The eating window should be of 8 hours. However, you must try to limit the number of times you eat in these 8 hours. Intermittent fasting is all about managing the number of meals and hours, it doesn't lay very great emphasis on the things you eat. It is natural to expect anyone trying to lose weight to eat healthy things. So, you should avoid eating fast food and food items rich in refined sugar. Most processed items or so-called low-fat food products are high on sugar. You should try to avoid them. But, you don't need to count calories if you are eating healthy things.

The Breakfast

This should be the heaviest meal of the day. You will be entering the most active phase of the day and would also be ending your fasting schedule. Therefore, it is very natural for you to feel very hungry. You can treat yourself with a good meal. However, the best tip for your breakfast meal would be to have a high-fat and low-carb diet. The fat gives more energy but is very slow to burn. This means that by having a high-fat diet, you will be able to go without food till your lunch effortlessly. You wouldn't feel the urge to have snacks in between and that is our goal.

The meals high in carb get digested very fast. They provide instant energy but would make you feel hungry very soon. It is best to avoid such items that are very high in carbs. The protein should be the second most important part of your meal after fat. You should consume moderate amounts of protein. It also takes longer to get processed, and it is very important for building muscles. However, you must avoid overdoing protein as that would do no good to you. If your diet is too high on protein, it would also start adding too many calories.

Therefore, 65-75% of the calories from your meals should come from fat, around 20% of the calories should come from protein, and only 5-10% of the calories should come from carbs.

The carbs that eat should only be things that are rich in fiber. It means you should only try to eat whole grain foods, non-starchy green leafy vegetables and things like that which have very high digestive fiber content.

The Lunch

It is the second meal of the day, and you should try to keep it very healthy. Eating fiber-rich food items like salads and fruits is always the best as it keeps you feeling light and fresh. A very heavy lunch often makes people feel drowsy.

The Dinner

This should be the lightest and healthiest meal of the day. People have a misconception that if they don't eat much in the dinner, they won't be able to make it through the fasting window easily. This has no basis. In fact, if you have a very heavy dinner, you are most likely to face problems like indigestion and food cravings.

This meals should be rich in digestive fiber. The digestive fiber takes very long to get processed while it adds very few calories to your system. This would mean that you will not feel hungry for very long after having your dinner.

If you are a morning person, never try to start your fasting late at night.

The more you delay the time of the fast, the longer you would have to remain in the fasted state in the morning. That is mostly very difficult for people.

The 16:8 Fasting for the Late Nighters

If you are a person who likes to burn the midnight oil, then beginning your fasting early in the evening wouldn't be such a great idea for you. However, this shouldn't mean that you can have it around midnight. Always try to time the beginning of your fasting window 4-5 hours prior to your bed-time. Going to bed immediately after having dinner can be very bad for your health.

You can have your dinner around 9 pm so that you can have your first meal of the day at noon. Everything else remains the same.

Intermittent fasting doesn't impose any hard and fast rule on you. The way you want to manage your food and lifestyle would always be up to you. However, it is expected of you to follow strict eating and fasting windows as they help in the regulation of your insulin levels, hGH, ghrelin, leptin, and several other hormonal levels. The timing is also very important for ensuring the good health of your digestive system and other vital organs.

The 16:8 intermittent fasting is the easiest to follow as it can be turned into a schedule. Your body adapts to its routine very quickly and times the feasting and fasting patterns. It is a very easy and sustainable way to live your life. You can make it a part of your life and may never feel the need to change it. It doesn't require you to make any other significant change in your lifestyle other than changing the hours you remain in the fasted state. It is simply like shifting your breakfast time a bit farther.

It is the best intermittent fasting schedule for all those people who have been repenting their inability to pay any special attention to their health. All those people who regretted their inability to take time out for exercise, diets, and meal planning can follow this routine and have all the health advantages with minimum effort. The 8 hours of eating window gives you complete freedom to eat literally anything as long as you are showing responsible behavior and reasonable restraint.

So, if you had been cursing your increasing weight, abdominal fat, and inability to do anything about it, this fasting routine gives you the chance you had been waiting for.

The Warrior Fasting- 20:4 Fasting Protocol

As the name suggests, this fasting schedule is for the people who have the warrior spirit. First, let us understand the significance of its name.

Our ancestors lived the lives of warriors. In fact, for every meal, a war was fought. Their food was the biggest foe. The animals they preyed upon were faster, stronger, and more capable than them. Getting food was uncertain, and most people traveled far to get their prey.

This meant that the probability of getting food was generally once in a day. The Braves went in search of food and when they returned with the prize, the whole group could have food only after that. This led to natural longer fasting. However, eating only once a day didn't make them weak. On the contrary, science has proven that your mind becomes more focused when your body has been running without food for around 24 hours. The physical instincts also get sharper. You are able to respond better and react faster. These were the abilities that helped them to hunt the animals which were better equipped than them. Fasting for longer increases the adrenaline rush in your body, and your stamina increases. You are able to endure fatigue better and test the physical limits of your body.

The same lifestyle is the inspiration for the 20:4 intermittent fasting schedule. The warrior fasting is the most popular schedule for bodybuilders and people involved in performance sports. It helps them in increasing their stamina and strength. They can do their workouts for longer and have a good supply of natural hGH and adrenaline in their blood. This is the reason they are able to achieve such extreme levels of low body fat and high muscle mass. They train for hours at end and don't face severe exhaustion.

The Process

The warrior fasting requires you to continue your fasting state for 20 hours at a stretch. Although it may look like that 4 hours is enough to fit two meals, but they aren't. It is very unlikely to have a second meal within such a short gap especially when you have consumed a very heavy meal with a lot of fat, protein, and very little carb. So effectively, 20:4 fasts mean one meal a day. You can have an elaborate single meal over a broad course which should start with lighter things like soup and then have the real food after a while once your body starts feeling a bit nourished.

Ending a long fast with a very heavy or solid meal is never advisable as it doesn't give your body the time to adjust. Always get off the fast with something light and then get on to heavier stuff. Therefore, the 4 hours given in this schedule are purely for having a simple big meal distributed over a considerably long period.

You can start your fasting whenever you want as there is no way to pass the whole fasting window in the dormant state. However, it best to time most of your workout schedule at the end of the fasting window as the production of hGH and adrenaline would be at its peak by the end. It will help in faster bulking of muscles. You would be able to work out harder and better.

The eating window is also very important as your energy demands would increase significantly, and you would have a considerably short span to consume all the required calories. Your warrior diet must consist of high-fat and high protein diet with very low or no carbohydrates. All the carbohydrates that you consume must only come from non-starchy green leafy vegetable and salads as they only supply fiber and very few calories. High-fat food would help you in going strong for the next 20-22 hours without food as they can provide energy for long. Fat takes a very long time to get processed and keeps you feeling satiated.

Switching to a high-fat diet and long fasting also starts the fat burning process in your body. It means your body starts using your own body fat for producing energy if you have high-fat content. This is a great intermittent fasting routine for all those people who can fit the bill.

However, you should never begin your tryst with intermittent fasting from this as then your chances of failure would increase considerably. This is a pro-routine which requires a great deal of practice and discipline. This routine is very hard to turn into a sustainable habit. It has to be followed strictly as a bulking routine. The warrior routine has several other health advantages too apart from fat loss and muscle buildup.

- It is a very helpful routine for stabilizing your blood sugar levels.
- You will feel more energetic and active.
- It is especially very helpful in improving your cognitive function.
- Warrior fasting is also very helpful in reducing chronic inflammations

It should only be carried out in weekly cycles.

Eat-Stop-Eat Method

This intermittent fasting method involves remaining in a complete fasting state continuously for 24 hours at least twice in a week on non-consecutive days. It means you can fast for a full 24 hours and then eat normally the next day. On the eating days must apply great restraint and not eat unhealthy things or not eat excessively. Then you can fast on any other day in the week in the same manner.

This is a simple and easy to understand intermittent fasting schedule. There are no extra rules. You only need to fast for 24 hours on two separate days of your choice in any given week. During your fasting days, you can have black tea, coffee, green tea, and fresh lime as long as they are unsweetened. As long as you are not adding sugar to these things, they will not break your fast and provide a lot of antioxidants.

These longer fasts have a very positive impact on your health. Besides all other specific advantages that come with intermittent fasting, these fasts also help by initiating the amazing process of "Autophagy."

Although this routine gives you great flexibility to fast on the days of your choice and does not impose the restriction of fasting every day, it is difficult to follow as a routine. Due to the longer duration of the fasts and the long gap in the fasting days, it becomes almost impossible to make them a normal habit for your body. You are most likely to feel the hunger pangs on the days of the fast. Following this routine on a regular basis makes it a bit easy but that doesn't change the fact that your body would go through the churning. However, the stress exerted by this routine is very positive and gives great results.

Alternate Day Fasting—24-Hour Fasting Protocol

Alternate day fasting is also similar to eat-stop-eat intermittent fasting routine in most respects, the only difference being that it is more regular in nature. It means that you will have to follow the fasting and eating days every other day. It means that there will be fasting days when you will have to remain without food for the complete duration of 24 hours. You can eat normally for the next 24 hours in which you will maintain a healthy diet. The next 24 hours will again be observed as the fasting hours, again followed by a day of feasting normally.

This can definitely be a very taxing routine as you will have to observe fasting every other day. However, a good thing about this routine is that it is considerably easy to make it a routine. Although your body would never take 24-hour fasts to be a norm, yet the hunger pangs subside after a period of time, and you are better able to remain in the fasted state.

This routine has amazing health advantages, and it starts running the process of autophagy at a much better speed. You can get visible anti-aging effects and feel much younger in appearance as well as the energy levels.

However, you must remember that this fasting method is not for beginners. Fasting every other day for someone who is not used to fasting schedules is neither easy not suitable. You must first practice the easier routine and only try this once your body has got used to the fasting stress.

The Fast Diet—5:2 Diet Protocol

This is an interesting inclusion in the list as it is not a fasting protocol in the real terms. It is more of a calorie restrictive regime, but it has shown great promise and results and that has inspired me to include this in the list.

It is one of the easiest ways to lose weight and has been very effective for women as it prevents any kind of hormonal imbalance that may occur due to fasting for longer hours.

This protocol involves eating normally within the specified calorie range for 5 days of the week and following a calorie restricted diet on two non-consecutive days of the week when the calorie consumption needs to be brought very low.

For men, the permissible calorie intake on the fasting days should be 600 calories. However, there is no restriction on the number of meals in which you can consume these calories. You only need to ensure that you do not cross this calorie threshold. If you can reasonably divide 600 calories into 3 meals, then this method doesn't object to it.

For women, the permissible calorie limit is 500 in a day. It means that through the course of the whole day, women can consume 500 calories at the most.

This method has been very effective in controlling weight and improving several health biomarkers.

Spontaneous Meal Skipping

This is also not a form of intermittent fasting but a way to increase the gap between your meals so that you can get the benefits of intermittent fasting without having to put up with the routine.

This method says that you must skip your meals whenever you are not feeling really hungry. It is an obvious thing to do if you look at it reasonably. However, you will be surprised if you reconsider your own eating patterns. We all have become so habitual of routines that we do most of the things out of the force of habit. It means when the clock strikes 1-2 in the afternoon and it is officially declared as the lunchtime, you have your lunch. Most of the times, it isn't the hunger that forces you to have lunch but simply a habit.

We also indulge ourselves in impulsive eating when we see others having something or have a food stall in front of us. Those are the times when we aren't hungry at all but still grab a bite. These are extra calories going into your system that can never be used. They are bound to get stored as fat.

Spontaneous meal skipping inspires you to only have a meal when you are actually feeling hungry. If you are not feeling a strong urge to eat, you must skip the meal and not cave in under the pressure of time or habit.

This meal skipping will help your body in developing insulin sensitivity and improve overall health biomarkers.

Chapter 5: Things That Can Help in Making Your Intermittent Fasting More Effective

There are several things that can help your weight loss efforts and health gain efforts while you are following intermittent fasts.

Four important things that can especially boost your efforts are:

1. Balanced Food
2. Good Exercise
3. Adequate Sleep
4. Healthy Routine

We will be discussing the impact of good exercise and the ones to follow in a later chapter, and hence we will be skipping that part in this chapter. It will suffice here to mention that exercise can boost the health benefits of intermittent fasting several times.

Balanced Food

Food is an important part of our lives. We become what we eat. If you look closely, 90% of your physique is simply a result of the things you eat and the manner in which you eat it. This means that even if you are not pumping iron for hours in a gym, you can have a considerably good physique if you are eating balanced food.

The concept of balanced food has been misunderstood to a very great extent. Healthy and balanced food which will have all the required macronutrients. It should have the required amounts of micronutrients, vitamins, and minerals too.

The 3 Macronutrients for Your Good Health

Fat

Fat has been the most essential part of our diet since the very beginning. Our ancestors had no idea of farming. They could only hunt and gather. The things they killed to eat had a good amount of fat and protein. These two things are our basic requirements, and we got them through the meat. This is a reason we survived without difficulty. Even today, most carnivorous animals survive only on fat and protein.

The fat has several crucial functions to perform. It can provide you with long-lasting energy as it is slow burning fuel. Even small amounts of fat can give you energy for long. It packs a punch when it comes to the number of calories in a specific amount of food. Fat has almost double the calories as compared to carbs in weight.

You can eat more fat at a time and store more energy while you will eat the same amount of carbs and get less energy. Fat also provides insulation against cold. It was also a reason our ancestors needed fat so much as fur coats and other clothing material was not at their disposal.

It is a macronutrient that must be a part of your weight loss diet.

There is a general misconception created by the food producing industry that eating fat would make you fat. There is nothing more absurd than this theory. Whatever you eat gets converted into energy in one or the other form. Therefore, fat making you fat and carbs not doing the same has no basis. However, the phobia from fat led to low-fat foods. People are crazy about low-fat foods and that has caused more obesity than anything else.

When fat is taken out of anything, not only the fat goes away but also the things that make the food tasty. Low-fat foods will not have any taste. The food industry can't sell tasteless food and therefore, it adds a lot of refined sugar in various forms to compensate for the loss of taste, and this increases the problem several times. Sugar adds more empty calories, causes cravings, leads to inflammations in the liver and spikes your insulin levels.

Your food must be rich in fat. In fact, 65-75% of the calories you consume in a day must come from fat. High-fat food would ensure that you are able to withstand long intervals between your meals easily. It also helps in beginning the process of ketosis.

Ketosis is the process of burning the ketones in your body. When your body is devoid of glucose energy, it has no other option than to burn the fat.

Your body is equipped to run on both kinds of fuel i.e. glucose and fat. However, it can't run on both at the same time. Now, glucose derived from the carbs is an easy to burn fat and therefore your body prefers to burn it. But it can run on fat if it is devoid a high carb diet.

When you are consuming a high-fat diet with moderate levels of protein and very low levels of carbs, your body starts burning fat for energy and this process is called ketosis.

It is one of the best diets for a person trying to lose weight and fat. This kind of diet is called the Ketogenic diet or the Keto diet. We will be discussing it in detail ahead.

Protein

Protein is important for your body as you need it for building muscles. Every day you lose some muscles and build new ones. For building new muscles, you will need to eat protein as it is the building block of muscles. However, you should only eat protein in moderate quantities as excessive protein would also be converted to blood sugar which you would want to avoid.

The ideal percentage of protein in your diet should be 15-20%. It means of all the calories that you get, only 15-20% calories should come from protein. Lean meats, egg whites, fish, cereals, kidney beans, and several nuts are great sources of protein.

Carbohydrate

Carbs are the primary source of energy we are consuming these days. Most of the weight gain issues faced these days are due to high consumption of carbs. However, projecting all types of carbs as the villain is not correct.

If you are consuming refined carbs then you are definitely going to invite trouble as these carbs get digested very fast and give an instant boost of energy. However, they cannot provide you with energy in the long term or keep you feeling satisfied. Therefore, eating such carbs would lead to food cravings. Sugar laced products also do the same. They add empty calories to your system and cause a great insulin spike. Your body gets a sudden energy kick but nothing for your gut to process. This can act very bad on your digestive process.

However, there are good carbs too. The carbs that you get from whole grains like barley, maze, and other such whole grains contain several important trace minerals that are essential for your body. You need these minerals, and these carbs are a great source. Then whole grain crabs also add a lot of digestive fiber to your system. This fiber plays a very important role in the health of your digestive system.

The fiber helps in cleaning the digestive system as it cannot be digested. It keeps your gut busy for very long, and hence you keep feeling satisfied even with small amounts of meals.

You also get a lot of soluble fiber, vitamins, minerals, and antioxidants from non-starchy green leafy vegetables. You can eat them as much as you want without being conscious about the calorie measurements. They are very healthy, and the soluble fiber forms a gel-like substance in your gut which helps in treating most of the digestive tract issues. The vitamins, minerals, & antioxidants in these vegetables also help you in staying healthy.

If you want to lose weight, the portion of carbohydrates in your diet should be very small. This is not including the non-starchy green leafy vegetables as you can consume them as much as you want. You should limit the intake of carbs from other things and only consume carbs in the form of whole grains and vegetables.

The calorie contribution of carbs should not be more than 5-10% and all of it must come from whole grains and vegetables.

Good Exercise

Exercise is important as it helps you in burning the fat faster. Exercise helps you in creating an extra energy demand. However, as your body is in the fasting state during your exercise, it cannot fulfill that energy demand by burning glucose. This forces your body to burn fat for producing energy and fat burning takes place. This process is very simple, but it cannot take place if your body has a ready supply of glucose. In that case, you will only be burning that glucose energy without disturbing your fat stores ever.

Therefore, it is important that you do all your exercises and especially the high-intensity interval training exercises at the end of your intermittent fasting schedules. This is the time when your fat burning abilities are at their peak.

Adequate Sleep

Giving your body the required amount of rest and sleep is also very important as it helps in proper recovery from the light positive stress caused by fasting and exercise. It is very important that you never ignore this aspect.

Sleep has some very crucial roles to play in your health.

1. The production of the hGH is at its peak while you are sleeping, and it helps in fat burning

2. Your body can produce high amounts of adrenaline in your sleep that will boost your performance
3. Your body carries out a lot of repair and rejuvenation work while you sleep. If your sleep is not adequate, these activities can get affected
4. Lack of sleep can make your body release stress hormones like cortisol. These hormones can stop any kind of fat burning as they push your body in the same mode. If you want to lose weight and remain healthy, proper sleep is a must for you.

Healthy Routine

Following a healthy routine is very important for the smooth functioning of your body. Intermittent fasting is a routine, and the word "routine" is very important here. It is not something that you can one day or one week and you will be able to reap the benefits for your whole life.

Your body goes through changes every day. It faces the challenges every day and therefore, it needs to be treated well on a regular basis. If you are following the intermittent fasting schedule on an irregular basis, you will not be able to stay healthy and fit.

The reason for the great success of intermittent fasting also lies in this very fact that it is a very sustainable way of living life. You can integrate the intermittent fasting in your life and may never need to change anything in your schedule. Therefore, if you want to lead a healthy life, you must make intermittent fasting a routine.

It is also important to have a healthy and active lifestyle. Our weight depends on the simple calculation of the number of calories consumed minus the number of calories burned. If you are living a sedentary lifestyle, you will not be burning any more extra calories than the ones burned by your metabolic processes and fat accumulation would get faster.

Stress is also a big reason for most of the health concerns. The higher the stress you take, the more you are likely to engage in emotional eating and other such activities that also lead to weight gain. If you are facing high-stress or any other kind of emotional turbulence in your life, you must try to deal with it immediately.

Chapter 6: Intermittent Fasting and Keto

Advantages of Keto on Intermittent Fasting

Intermittent fasting and keto diet are a match made in heaven. Both initiate the same process and work towards bringing the same results. The Keto diet involves increasing the fat in your food to the highest levels with moderate proteins and no or very low carbs.

This helps your body in running on fat fuel as the supply of glucose fuel is blocked completely. So, either you are consuming food or burning your body fat, the process remains the same, and the body doesn't have to make the switch frequently. This one thing makes both the processes so compatible.

When you begin your intermittent fasting, you force your body to burn the body fat by cutting off glucose supply. However, if you are on a normal diet, your body would again switch back to burning glucose provided by the carbs. It doesn't happen in case of a keto diet as through food also you get only fat.

Your body starts the effective process called the ketosis. When your body is not getting energy from any other source, the fat cells start releasing the ketones. These ketones can be converted into energy. This process of burning the ketones is called ketosis.

At the beginning of intermittent fasting, people can face several side effects as your body goes through sugar withdrawal symptoms. These symptoms can be a feeling of light-headedness, nausea, and weakness. Although these symptoms are temporary, some people get really worried. Combining intermittent fasting with a ketogenic diet can help you in suppressing some of these symptoms too.

Another big advantage of ketosis is fat oxidation. When your body is constantly burning glucose fuel, it releases a lot of by-products known as AGEs that promote chronic inflammation and oxidative stress.

The tumors in the body are also affected if you are on a keto diet. Actually, the scientists have recently found that the only difference between the functioning of tumor cells of your body and the normal cells is that they cannot survive on energy provided by the fat-rich diet. They lack the components that can metabolize fat. This means if you are on a keto diet, you can literally starve the cells causing and spreading cancer and tumors in your body. All the other normal cells in our body can metabolize fat and therefore, they won't get affected.

You would feel less hungry while on a keto diet. The fat can keep you feeling satisfied for much longer.

Some of the Best Foods to eat while on a Keto Diet:

1. Seafood
2. Non-starchy green leafy vegetables
3. Cheese
4. Avocados
5. Meat and Poultry
6. Eggs
7. Coconut Oil
8. Olive Oil
9. Cottage Cheese and Yogurt
10. Nuts and Seeds
11. Berries
12. Butter
13. Shirataki Noodles
14. Olives
15. Black tea and coffee
16. Dark Chocolate

There might be some symptoms that will show that your body has begun the process of ketosis.

Main Signs Telling Your Ketosis Has Begun

Bad Breath

The level of ketones increases in your blood when your body starts ketosis. This can give your breath a fruity smell. It should indicate that your diet is working for you.

High Ketones in Your Blood Work

Although you will not get to know this change without a blood test if you are following a keto diet and want to know if you have entered ketosis, you can take a blood test. High levels of ketones in your blood will be a testimony to the fact that ketosis has started.

Low Appetite

Once your body enters ketosis, you will notice suppression in your appetite. Your urge to eat will go away. There is no reason to worry about this. It happens because your body starts using a long-lasting fuel. Its need to consume food for short term energy ends. Even if you are not eating anything, the body manages to run its energy supply by burning your body fat and that's why you feel less hungry.

Better Focus and Energy

Fat is a clean fuel and provides cleaner energy without leaving less toxic waste. There is low oxidative stress, and other problem items like the VLDLs and triglycerides are also getting used along with free fatty acids. This leads to cleaner energy. Your brain also starts using this energy and works better. This leads to better focus and high energy.

Fatigue in the Initial Stages

This is a side-effect most people face in the initial stages and worry about. However, there is nothing to worry about. It happens when your body is adjusting to the change in the fuel burning mechanism. If you are feeling the fatigue too much, you should try taking electrolytes. They help in suppressing the symptoms. You should also take sodium, potassium, and magnesium supplements in your daily diet.

Diarrhea and Constipation

These are the real problems that some people face and there is no getting around these problems. Your digestive system has to make a lot of changes when you shift from carbs rich diet to a keto diet. This may lead to these issues. However, these symptoms are also temporary and go away very soon.

Sleep Issues

Sleep issues can become a problem in the initial stages of starting a keto diet. Although this problem is temporary, some people can get restless as they are unable to sleep properly. However, there is no reason to worry as your body would soon adjust, and you will have much better sleep that earlier.

Fat and Weight Loss

There is no doubt in the fact that fat and weight loss is among the most notable symptoms of entering ketosis. The impact of ketosis is visible in your appearance. You would rapidly lose weight and would start to measure less around your waist circumference. This is one sign that you would love.

Chapter 7: Exercise and Intermittent Fasting

Exercise is a sure-shot way to increase the benefits of intermittent fasting. It helps in faster fat burning and also promotes muscle buildup. You can improve your stamina by doing regular exercise and improve your body's response against stress, especially of your heart.

When you do high-intensity interval training, a nitric oxide dump takes place which can catalyze and promote health. It soothes your muscles and helps them in relaxing. This can be crucial for organs like a heart which are generally under high stress.

When you are at the end of your fasting cycle, the production of hGH and adrenaline is at its peak. This hormone can enhance your abilities to do exercise.

Exercise also helps in improving the way in which muscles repair themselves. You can have a faster rate of recovery from injuries if you exercise regularly.

Exercise is also very important if you want to burn your fat faster. It increases the energy demands of your body. Hence, the body has no other option than to burn fat to produce that required energy. This leads to faster fat burning.

Although exercise is one of the best ways to speed up the results of intermittent fasting, some important rules need to be followed. For instance, if you are following longer fasts, then you should avoid doing high-intensity interval training (HIIT) on the days of your fasts. This is due to the reason that your body is in an energy deficit mode, and you may start feeling tired pretty soon.

You must also avoid doing HIIT on consecutive days. This is to prevent overstressing your body. HIIT puts a lot of strain on your body and especially the muscles for which you have done exercise. Doing the same exercises on consecutive days will put an extra burden on those muscles. A lot of muscles break and regenerate after exercise. Continuous stress can cause injuries. There must be days of rest between your exercise days. It will give your muscles the time to recover.

Best Ways to Exercise

HIIT

High-intensity Interval Training (HIIT) is one of the best ways to make your body burn fat. You can get faster results by investing little time in HIIT. You may have to walk for much longer to get the same results which you can get from small sprints. It also helps in the better buildup of muscles.

On alternate days, do easy cardio exercises. You cannot do HIIT every day. However, on the days you are not doing HIIT, you must do light cardio exercises, yoga, brisk walking, etc. as these activities help you in staying fit. They are good for your heart health and also provide great relief.

You can do weight training on all days if you like as your body wouldn't need to put in much energy effort into that.

Give Your Body Time to Re-energize

This is very important. If you put a lot of stress on your body, it can have adverse effects on your health. Always start slow when you begin your intermittent fasting and then build your stamina as you move ahead.

Walk a Lot

People generally undermine the health benefits of brisk walks as they believe it doesn't lead to weight loss or fat burning. This is a misconception that needs to be broken. In fact, walking has several health benefits:

NEAT Also Uses Up Energy: When you walk or move around even for some time, your body consumes energy. It is like informal consumption of energy coming in short bursts. People do not count it as substantial, but it is. You can burn a lot of energy in this way and it will lead to weight loss.

Helps You in Suppressing Hunger: If you are feeling hungry or your mind is racing towards the thoughts of food, you must go for a short walk. It can help in suppressing hunger for good.

Good for Heart: Brisk walks are very good for the heart. They help in supplying oxygen in good amounts to the vital organs.

Chapter 8: Supplements

Intermittent fasting is a comprehensive solution for most of the health issues. However, when you start following any kind of routine that changes your eating patterns or the amount of food you eat, your body can get deficient in some nutrients. Nutrient supplements can help you in compensating for these deficiencies.

Drink Plenty of Fluids

While you are following intermittent fasting, your body will be a lot of detoxification. It means it will start cleansing itself. It will dump a lot of fluid, and with fluids, a lot of minerals are also lost. This is the biggest loss that happens, and you need to be careful about it.

The first thing that you must do is drink a lot of fluids. However, you should avoid drinking plain water or any kind of soda. The lost fluid had a lot of minerals, and when you drink a lot of plain water, the mineral levels in your body goes down. To prevent any kind of dehydration, you must always mix a pinch of sea salt to your water and it can help you.

Electrolytes

You can also drink electrolytes as they also help in preventing dehydration. You will not feel weak or dehydrated if you are consuming a lot of electrolytes.

Lime

Another way to prevent problems and keep yourself well hydrated is to have unsweetened fresh lime water with a pinch of sea salt. While doing intermittent fasting, it is important that you consume at least one fresh lime a day. You can use it for preparing fresh lime and that would also do the trick. This simple thing can prevent the formation of stones. Actually, when you start fasting, your body starts washing out calcium and other mineral deposits. Some of these minerals can accumulate as stones. Having a lime a day helps you in clearing out these substances from your body.

Potassium

Potassium is also an important mineral that you would need to take. You can get this mineral through natural sources like banana which has a lot of potassium. Pomegranate also has a lot of potassium, or you can also take potassium supplements.

It is important to keep your potassium levels up as it is an important mineral needed by your body. While you are doing intermittent fasting, your body is going through a lot of changes. It changes its fuel source and the way it was functioning. Potassium deficiency can increase problems.

Antioxidants

Chronic inflammations are one of the biggest villains when it comes to poor health. They keep weighing you down and you don't even get to know about them until it is very late. Intermittent fasting plays an important role in preventing chronic inflammations. You can also help in this cause by consuming food items that are high in antioxidants.

Healthy fats, nuts, seafood, vegetables, whole spices, turmeric, and garlic are some of the things which are high in antioxidants. You can take the antioxidants to speed up the healing process of your body. Antioxidants also play a very important role in preventing chronic inflammations.

B Vitamins

B vitamins are necessary, and you can't have enough of them. Taking these vitamins helps in promoting overall health.

Probiotic Foods

Your gut plays a very important role in promoting your health. However, it remains neglected most of the time, and we only pay any attention to it when there are problems related to our gut. Our gut has trillions of helpful bacteria that facilitate digestion of food and healthy digestive tract. However, overeating, acidity, gastric issues, bad foods, and antibiotics are some of the things that can cause great damage to these bacteria. You can help in repopulation of these bacteria by consuming probiotic food.

Magnesium

It is a mineral that our body needs for performing several crucial functions. It is a cofactor for hundreds of enzymes. We can get it from the vegetable green, but most people are usually deficient in magnesium as they don't consume vegetable greens. Its deficiency can affect your blood pressure, heart rhythm, muscle tone, vitamin D absorption, and stress. You can increase your intake of vegetable green for improving the magnesium levels or you can also take supplements to fulfill the deficiency.

Chapter 9: Intermittent Fasting for Women

Intermittent fasting is a great way to reduce weight and that's why it is always a reason for inquiry for women. Women are usually more conscious about their weight and looks than men. They want to lose weight faster and that's why the highest percentage of subscribers to fitness programs are women.

Intermittent fasting has also caught their attention and that's a reason most women start following intermittent fasting without proper research.

Following Intermittent Fasting Like Men Can Be Dangerous for Women

There is no other way to emphasize this fact more clearly. Yes, it is right. If women start following intermittent fasting like men, they can get into a lot of trouble. The reason lies in their own body. Women have a very sensitive hormonal system that can become overreactive if women start remaining hungry for very long without taking proper precaution.

Can Women Practice Intermittent Fasting?

Of course, they can practice intermittent fasting, and it can have a great impact on their weight. The only thing is that they need to take more precautions than usual. If they start keeping fasts without following precautions, their hormones get off the chart and start giving trouble. They are very sensitive to food. Women may hate to accept it, but the food is not only their physiological need but it also offers emotional and psychological assurances.

The Reasons for the Difference

The reason women need to follow intermittent fasting differently lies in the fact that they have different physiology. Nature has given them the gift of bringing another life into this world in the form of babies. This gift also requires them to be prepared for bearing a child at all times. Their bodies are more sensitive to fat accumulation, and they also have a sensitive hormonal system that reacts adversely to hunger. It means various hormones in the body of a women can go off the charts if a woman starts staying hungry for long all of a sudden.

Nature has made women in such a way that their bodies function better at a higher level of fat in the body as compared to men. Men should ideally have 10-15% of body fat, and they can function optimally at these levels. However, women need around 18–20% of body fat.

Their hormonal system is also very different. A woman's body bears a child. Most of the process of formation of a child takes place with the help of fat. This makes their bodies a bit protective of fat. Besides that, women can start feeling cranky, irritated, hyper, depressed, angry, and many other such things if they go hungry for long. This is also due to the way in which their hunger hormone ghrelin reacts with other hormones in their body.

This makes it necessary that women do not start any kind of drastic fast, calorie restrictive regimen, or diet without proper preparation and precautions.

Precautions for Women Who Want to Follow Intermittent Fasting

- Women who want to follow intermittent fasting must keep some important things in mind:
- Never begin fasting with any strict or longer fast
- Always give their body the time to adjust to the fasting schedules
- They shouldn't test the limits of endurance of their bodies as far as remaining hungry is concerned

- They should take supplements as loss of minerals can have a prominent impact on their health

Things to Remember

- If you want to follow intermittent fasting, always start with the simplest fast.
- Start by skipping the snacks first and then start increasing the time between meals.
- First, you must ensure that all your meals end within 12 hours window and start by practicing 12 hours fast.
- Once your body gets used to 12-hour fasts, you can start the 14:10 fasts.
- Always remain on a specific fasting routine for at least a fortnight before moving on to the next one.
- The 14:10 fasting schedule works best for women. It is neither too long nor short and gives great results.
- Women can also follow the 5:2 fasting protocol as it has also shown to benefit women a lot.
- Women should never keep a fast longer than 24 hours in any condition.
- While men are said to have benefited greatly from longer fasts, they have had adverse results on women.

When to Stop

It is very important that women must know when to stop intermittent fasting. Despite taking all the precautions, a woman's body may not react favorably to intermittent fasting. It can happen due to various reasons, and the biggest one is the different needs of every woman's body. A woman can react completely in a unique manner due to different stimuli. So, if you notice anything abnormal, then you must stop intermittent fasting and consult a physician immediately.

Given below are some of the conditions in which women should immediately stop intermittent fasting.

If Trying to Conceive

If you are trying to have a child, then you must immediately stop intermittent fasting or following any kind of calorie restrictive regimen. Several studies have shown that fasting or depriving the body of food and nutrients for long can cause fertility organs to shrink temporarily. Therefore, if you are trying to conceive, it may take much longer to get successful or you may not be able to conceive at all as long as you are on fasts.

On Getting Pregnant

If you have gotten pregnant, you must stop intermittent fasting immediately. A pregnant woman has very high energy needs. She is making a baby out of the body fat and also needs to nurture the baby with the energy she gets from the food she consumes. Therefore, she should stop intermittent fasting immediately.

While Nursing

If you are nursing a child, you shouldn't follow intermittent fasting for that duration as it may lead to nutrient deficiency. Your body needs more energy and for that, you need to eat properly.

If the Periods Become Erratic

Some women may have erratic menstrual periods due to calorie deprivation. If anything like that happens, you may need to adjust your fasting periods. If the problem persists, you must consult a physician immediately.

If There Are Sudden Changes in Eating Patterns

The eating patterns of some women can get affected adversely due to longer fasting periods. They may stop feeling hungry or may keep feeling famished. If the problems are minor, they must make an adjustment in their eating patterns. However, if the problem is serious a physician must be consulted immediately.

Other Signs Indicating That You Should Stop Intermittent Fasting

- On continuously feeling cold
- When facing acute digestion issues for long
- When you start feeling weak in the heart or have feelings of palpitation
- When the mood swings become very frantic and erratic
- If your skin has started to appear very dry all of sudden or you have developed acne
- If you start noticing sudden and significant hair fall for no apparent reason
- When you start having sleep issues
- When you become very averse to romance all of a sudden
- When your ability to bear the stress of any kind reduces significantly

Chapter 10: The Best Ways to Handle Hunger Pangs and Cravings

Hunger pangs and cravings can be tough to handle at times. When hunger pangs and cravings start taking control of your mind, the only thing that comes to mind is food. Your mind remains fixated, and the time starts to stretch for you. Passing even minutes seems like an hour. You remain seated at one place with your mind wandering around food. This is the times when your digestive system also starts its churning. You start getting a grumpy and growling stomach. To make matters worse, there can be an acute stomach ache. Headache and irritation can also come following all these symptoms. All this could happen because you are having a strong urge to eat. These are extreme scenarios, but they happen with everyone once a while.

However, if you start practicing intermittent fasting you will have to become a pro at handling hunger pangs and cravings for good as ignoring them can make you a regular victim of these problems.

Keep Yourself Busy

It is a very important thing that if you are sitting idle in the fasting period, you will feel stronger hunger pangs, and your mind would wander around food more frequently. The best way to deal with this problem is to keep yourself busy. The more occupied your mind remains, the less it would think about food. Remember that most of the times when you are feeling the urge to eat anything, it is an excuse of your mind to create a diversion from current events or to avoid any work. So, hunger pangs can be easily avoided or tolerated if you are occupied with some work.

Keep Drinking Water

This one is also very important. Water is such a beautiful beverage. You can drink plenty of it and have no consequences. It will fill up your stomach without adding any calories. If you drink enough, you can make hunger go away easily. However, you must remember one important thing, do not drink too much water without adding a pinch of sea salt. Drinking too much plain water can lead to excessive urination, and it would drain you of minerals. So, either drink electrolytes, fresh life water without sugar or add a pinch of sea salt to your water and you can drink it safely.

Eat Fiber and Protein Rich Food

One of the best ways to help you feel satisfied without having unnecessary food cravings is to have a lot of fiber and good amounts of protein in your diet. Protein is heavy and takes time to get digested; this makes it sit in your stomach. Your stomach doesn't feel empty very fast, and you can go without feeling hungry for much longer. Eating fiber-rich food is also an easy and good way to avoid cravings for food. The fiber doesn't get digested and keeps your stomach busy for very long. Therefore, if you fear the cravings of food, then start eating food that is rich in protein and fiber.

Drink Unsweetened Black Tea and Coffee or Green Tea

Black tea, coffee, and green tea are some of the beverages that do not add any calories to your system and hence can be consumed safely during your fasting window. Apart from that, these beverages are rich in antioxidants and help you in fighting several problems. When you begin intermittent fasting, leave sugar, or start a keto diet, you can face symptoms like lightheadedness, weakness, nausea, headache, and other similar issues. These are temporary signs of sugar withdrawal. These beverages also help you in fighting these symptoms successfully.

Don't Remain Awake Until Late at Night

Sleep is very important when it comes to taking the full advantage of intermittent fasting. It helps in fighting various chronic issues, and your body is also able to fight stress and other problems. However, one more thing in which your sleep helps you is fighting hunger pangs. When you remain awake for too long, your brain starts playing with you and gives a feeling that you are hungry. It happens very often, and the best way to fight this feeling is to never stay awake till very late at night. In this way, you will not only be saving your body from overtaxing itself but also escape the hunger pangs.

Use Vanilla Scented Candles to Keep Cravings Away

If your cravings for sweet are very high and you keep feeling like eating sweets, the best way to fight that urge is to light vanilla scented candles in your room. These sweet-smelling candles reduce your cravings for sweets. It works in the fashion of incremental threat effect theory where overexposure to something leads to less likeliness of that thing.

Exercise

Exercise can also help you in distracting your mind from eating. Several hormones are released during exercise that helps you stay away from food. You feel more energized, and your mind also gets distracted.

Go for a Walk

This is also one of the best options to stay away from food. Walking gives your mind a healthy distraction from the thoughts of food. You get a chance to think about other things. It can help you in fighting the hunger pangs.

It is important to remember that hunger pangs are very short. Your stomach releases a hormone called ghrelin when it feels that there is a need for food. This hormone sends the signals to the brain and the brain directs you to have food. However, if you ignore this signal for some time, the ghrelin release would subside, and you would stop feeling hungry anymore. You may have personally witnessed this several times when you had been feeling hungry some time ago, but because it took time to get food, you stopped feeling hungry anymore. So, if you are feeling the hunger pangs and yet it isn't the time to eat, sit tight for a bit and the feeling would subside on its own.

Chapter 11: Ways to Stay Motivated

Weight loss may be a daunting task for which you may be prepared to go to any length. However, staying hungry is also not an easy task either. Most of the people are troubled by their weight when they are in public. Apart from those who have severe health issues, overweight people do not have much of an issue with their weight in close quarters. However, it is not the same as staying hungry. Either you are in public or all alone, staying hungry can make you anxious if you haven't conditioned your mind well. In some circumstances, you may even feel bothered when you are with others.

Pushing yourself to stay hungry and on track isn't an easy task. It is very easy to feel the urge to cheat once a while. However, once you give yourself the leeway, it is very difficult to get back and you see all your effort getting flushed down the drain which can be very sad and demotivating.

This is a battle easiest to fight when there is someone with whom you can share your ordeals or who can provide moral support and the required distraction when needed. If you have a support group, you can ask for advice, share your problems or just even discuss things related to your progress. There can be several ways to have this moral support in your life.

- You can share your journey with your close and understanding friends
- You can discuss your desires with your family
- With other people facing the same problems. You can work as an anchor for each other
- You can also join support groups
- Join online communities

Are Support Groups Really Important?

It depends upon your outlook, the kind of person you are, and the amount of weight you want to lose. If your weight loss targets are normal and you are not facing obesity in real terms, you may do fine even without support groups. If you live in a close-knit family, you may not need to find your moral support elsewhere. If you have close friends who care for you, then you would already have a support group.

However, if you are living alone or facing problems in sharing your concerns, thoughts, and worries, then the support groups may do more good to you than you can think. The support groups can not only provide sympathy and support but they also provide valuable advice, insights, and counseling. There can be several types of support groups to join.

Some Common Types of Support Groups Other Than Your Friends and Family

Commercial Programs

There can be several institutions running weight loss programs and counseling programs. They have their own set of experts who can suggest you better ways to follow your weight loss journey. There are experts to guide you on every step of the way, and hence the journey becomes easier. You have people to look up to and the ones with whom you can discuss the perils in the way.

The success rate of people in these groups is generally high as they find it easy to remain motivated. The experts in the group keep motivating these people and show them the way to move forward.

Enrolling in Clinic-Based Programs

This is a more professional approach to weight loss and other health issues. There are experts to monitor your progress and they keep guiding you on every step. It is always easy to get a professional answer to your queries, and the dangers of things going horribly wrong anywhere are very less as the people handling the progress are actually medical professionals. It is a bit expensive way, but it works, and it is especially very good for you if you are already facing any serious health risk like diabetes, heart problems, or other such issues. Supervision of a medical professional helps you in remaining confident that if anything starts going wrong, an expert is there to guide you.

Volunteer Programs

These programs are run by volunteers and hence they are generally free. Most such programs are conducted for obtaining results for some studies over control groups. These programs offer advice for free, but they monitor the subjects very closely and expect them to follow the set conditions rigorously. In case the subjects fail to meet the desired goals, they can be taken off the programs. Although sticking to these groups might look difficult, their success rates are very high as every subject get individual attention and monitoring. The changes are made from time to time to get the desired results.

It doesn't matter whether you enroll in any kind of professional support group or confide your journey in your friends and family, the important thing is to stick to the protocols and keep making the adjustments.

There will be times when you may find the going getting tough. However, it will still be important to keep going.

Remember, obesity isn't simply a cosmetic problem; it opens Pandora's box of problems.

Choosing to live with obesity is choosing to live a life of limitations. You will limit your mental, physical, and emotional abilities. You will make a compromise to live an insufficient life.

Getting obese can occur with anyone, but only those people will remain so who don't show the courage to fight with the problem. Obesity isn't an irreversible handicap, but it does make you less of a person if you stop fighting it.

It will bring a number of diseases which will limit your freedom to do things in life. You may choose to live with diabetes, but you will need to remember that you could have tried to avert it. The same goes for high blood pressure, heart diseases, chronic inflammations, and other lifestyle disorders.

Therefore, it is the best option to stand up for yourself and fight against the malice called obesity.

Healthy living is your right, and nothing can take it away from you if you are determined. Intermittent fasting is one of the easiest ways to fight this big enemy. The only thing required from you is to stay strong in the journey and face the enemy with full might.

Chapter 12: The Good, the Bad, and the Ugly of Intermittent Fasting

Every coin has two faces, and even intermittent fasting isn't an exception. Like every other method, there are some things that can trouble people practicing intermittent fasting. This chapter will explain the good, the bad, and the ugly of intermittent fasting. It will explain the symptoms that will go away very soon. It will also explain the problems which if persist, you may need to make changes. And finally, it will explain the things in the light of which, you must not follow intermittent fasting as that can be risky.

The Good

The good thing is that most of these troubles are temporary. Your body needs to go through some major changes, and the side effects that you may face will be a part of that change and hence, you will stop experiencing those symptoms very soon and hence, if you face them, there should be no reason to worry. You may find these issues to be difficult, but they are minor troubles and wouldn't affect you much in the long-run.

Cravings

Having strong cravings to eat sweets is a common problem people face in the initial stages of intermittent fasting. It would happen more if you continue eating sweets and sugar. These cravings can make you restless, but there is no need to panic as these symptoms will pass away very soon. Eating sweets lead to the release of certain chemicals that make you feel good. However, this feeling is short-lived, and as soon as it passes away, you want to eat more to feel that state of goodness. It is a vicious cycle and leads to no good. Eating sweets will continue adding empty calories to your system that would cause more harm. Therefore, even if you feel the cravings to eat sweet, you must avoid it, and soon, you will find that you don't want to eat sweets anymore.

Hunger Pangs

We have already discussed that hunger pangs are temporary, and the ways to deal with hunger pangs have also been discussed in the chapter earlier. Hunger pangs are temporary, and soon, your body will get used to staying in the fasted state for the set period easily.

Feeling Low

This is a problem that people feel initially. However, there is no reason to worry as this happens when your body is still learning to burn fat for energy. Our bodies have got used to glucose fuel, and they want to run it that way. It is a short-lived fuel and that's why you start feeling low soon after you have consumed your meal. Once your body gets adjusted to ketosis, you will stop feeling low on energy. On the contrary, you will feel more energetic and livelier.

Headache

Headaches are a part of the sugar withdrawal symptoms that would end very soon. You can take unsweetened black tea or coffee once or twice when you feel the headaches and soon after a few days of practicing intermittent fasting the headaches would go away.

Irritation

There can be a feeling of irritation for unknown reasons. It happens due to hunger and sugar cravings. However, the irritation would also not last very long, and you can try to divert your mind to other things to get over the temporary feelings of irritation.

Constipation or Diarrhea

When you start practicing intermittent fasting and keto diet, the food and eating pattern changes drastically. Eating at regular intervals and eating junk have become a part of our lives. However, when you change your diet, your gut takes some time to adjust to the changes. Constipation, diarrhea, bloating, and heartburn are temporary issues. In fact, after a few days of practicing intermittent fasting, you would notice that problems like acidity, constipation, and heartburn would vanish completely. You would be able to process the food very easily.

Feeling Cold

You may at times feel the pores of your fingers and toes to be getting very cold. There is no reason for you to be concerned from this as the problem occurs due to lack of ready energy. The glucose fuel travels easily, whereas it takes time for your body to start moving the fat from your adipose tissues to your pores. However, if your pores have started feeling cold, then it means that your body has started the process, and it will soon start working very efficiently.

Overeating

This is a problem most people face in the initial stages. When they get off the fasting window, they feel famished and eat a lot which may also cause discomfort. This is an adjustment you'll learn to make soon. You will have to follow a bit of restraint when you get off your fast. Overeating can leave you feeling bloated. There is no reason to overeat as your body is already producing energy from fat. To prevent eating more, you must eat slowly. The more time you'll take to eat a meal, the less you will be able to eat as your satiety hormone 'leptin' would send signals to your brain to stop eating. It takes some time for your brain to recognize that you are full, and therefore, if you are eating fast, the chances of overeating increase. Take your time to eat meals, and this problem can be prevented.

Frequent Trips to the Bathroom

You may need to go to the bathroom several times when you start intermittent fasting. This happens because the body starts the detoxification process in the initial stages. You must keep yourself hydrated and drink a lot of water with sea salt and fresh lime. You can also drink electrolytes to prevent the loss of minerals.

The Bad

Fluctuation in Sugar Levels

The blood sugar level fluctuations can be bad. If you are suffering from diabetes, you must consult your doctor in the loop so that your insulin dosage can be adjusted accordingly. In the initial stages, this can happen more. However, there is no permanent solution to this problem. Intermittent fasting is one of the best ways to bring insulin sensitivity, but a problem that has been building for long would take a bit longer to treat. If you are having severe fluctuations in your blood sugar levels, you must consult your doctor. Ignoring it can have serious health repercussions.

Constipation for Long

If the problem of constipation persists for long, you must consult a doctor. It can be due to some other issues too. Ignoring the problem as a normal symptom can be dangerous.

Any Persistent Problem

Most of the symptoms stated above should subside within a week or a fortnight. But, if any problem persists for longer than that, you must consult a doctor and try to find the real reason behind the problem. Intermittent fasting doesn't have any long-term side effect of this nature.

The Ugly

Developing Eating Disorders

This is a problem that some people can face. The chances are rare, but every person has a unique system, and some may react adversely to the changes. If you have had any eating disorders in the past, then you should avoid following intermittent fasting without consulting your doctor.

Persistent Problems Related to Health

If there is any health issue that you are facing despite taking all the care, then you should stop intermittent fasting and observe if the symptoms subside. If that happens, you should stop following intermittent fasting and ask for your doctor's advice.

Chapter 13: Myths and Misconceptions About Intermittent Fasting

Myths and misconceptions have an uncanny way of entering into the common belief. They have no basis, but they are repeated so many times that people start believing in them as truth. Every concept has been marred by these beliefs. Intermittent fasting is a proven way to reap a number of health benefits. You will be eating no pills that may cause side effects. You will not be subjecting yourself to any undue pressure that may cause any harm. Intermittent fasting is a simple way of improving your lifestyle and eating habits.

Given below are some common misconceptions about intermittent fasting that have no scientific basis.

Breakfast Is the Most Important Meal of the Day—Skipping It Will Make You Fat

This a statement every child grows up listening from parents, and it gets imbibed in the head as truth. Breakfast is the meal of the day which you take after breaking your nightly fast. There is nothing to prove that it needs to be early in the morning.

It is a fact that the first meal of the day should be heavy and balanced as it would help you in kickstarting your day. However, it can be taken at any time you like and having it early in the morning is not necessary.

As far as having a balanced and heavy breakfast is concerned, it is important. The reason is that you will be entering into the active part of the day with this meal. If you have a heavy and balanced breakfast, you will be able to push your cravings to have another meal as far as possible. If your breakfast is light, you may start feeling hungry very soon.

Pushing your breakfast to later part of the day will not have anything to do with your being fat. In fact, extending your fasting period will give you weight loss benefits.

You Must Eat Frequently to Keep Your Metabolism Running

This is a myth that has only benefitted the food manufacturing companies. Frequent meals have nothing to do with metabolism. The origin of this concept lies in the fact that your body uses up some energy in processing food. So, if you keep eating frequently, your metabolism will keep working and would burn more energy.

However, it doesn't take into account the fact that you will be consuming more energy than you will burn if you keep having meals at frequent intervals. The energy needed to metabolize the food is only 10–12% of the energy consumed. You will be piling up yourself by eating frequently.

Studies have clearly shown that people who follow intermittent fasting have up to 14% higher metabolism rate than those who don't.

Small Meals at Frequent Intervals Are Important for Losing Weight

This is also a continuation of the earlier myth and has no scientific basis. In fact, science has proven that the higher the number of meals, the greater would be fat storage would be as your insulin would keep storing the excess energy as fat. If you keep having meals at frequent intervals, your fat burning hormones will never be able to work at all.

Brain Will Stop Functioning Without Glucose

It is a fact that brain functions on glucose. However, it is a half baked truth that if you stop consuming carbs, your body would not have any other way to produce glucose. Your body has passed through thousands of years of evolutionary process. It makes no sense to believe that if one type of fuel source is cut off, it wouldn't be able to produce energy through other means.

Your body also has glycogen stores that can be used as energy. Then your body starts using ketones for energy, and your brain would never face a lack of energy to run itself. The brain is the most important organ of the body. It also controls all other functions in the body. It is also one organ that is made of pure fat. Your body serves your brain with complete devotion, and it would always supply it with the required energy either you consume carbs or not.

Our ancestors didn't have access to carbs. They solely relied on fat and protein. Their brains should have stopped functioning thousands of years ago if that was the case.

Your Body Will Enter the Starvation Mode if You Fast for Long

This is pure myth. Starvation mode is a survival mechanism of your body. Your body enters that starvation mode when it senses a complete energy supply cut off for very long. It takes 72-96 hours for the starvation mode to kick in. In this stage, your body lowers the metabolic rate and starts running only the crucial functions so that it can survive for the longest on the current energy reserves. The body of a healthy adult can run for months in starvation mode. For an obese person, this time can be even longer as the energy reserves are high.

However, the theory that starvation mode would kick in after short fasts have no scientific and reasonable basis. If that would have been the case, our ancestors wouldn't have survived for this long. They needed to be quicker and sharper after short fasting intervals as they needed to put more effort into catching the prey. Short fasts making them slow neither has evolutionary backing nor does it qualify on reason.

Studies have shown that after short fasts, your hGH levels can shoot up several times. In men, the hGH levels can rise up to 2000%, and in women, they can rise up to 1400%. The metabolic rate also goes up by 14%. The adrenaline production in your body also increases considerably. All these things show that you would be more alert, conscious, and active after short fasts.

You Will Lose Muscle Mass if You Follow Intermittent Fasting

People believe that fasting would start cannibalization of the muscles as soon as your blood glucose levels go down. This is a fear that also has no basis. It is a fact that your body first consumes the glucose and then it starts to look for a similar source like protein. However, it doesn't mean that it will eat up all the muscles. Muscles are important for survival your body knows better. Once your glucose supply ends, your body starts looking for alternative energy sources. Some damaged muscles can be used up but that is a part of the cleaning process. However, muscles cannot provide the kind of energy your body needs. It soon starts using fat stores for producing energy which is a steady and better source.

Some loss of muscles would take place with any kind of calorie restrictive regimen. However, the risk of this happening with intermittent fasting is a lot less as it forces and trains your body to burn fat. In fact, with the help of exercise, you can build more muscles than you lose. It is the main reasons that bodybuilders around the globe use intermittent fasting as a bulking routine.

Intermittent Fasting Will Lead to Binge Eating

This a problem that people face more with other diets and calorie restrictive routines than they with intermittent fasting.

Intermittent fasting puts no specific restriction on the number of calories you can eat or even the type of things you can eat. Therefore, the chances of temptation building and cravings are low. You always have the option to eat almost anything in your feasting window as long as you remain in a limit.

This isn't the case with people on diets and calorie restrictive routines as they severely limit the number of calories that can be consumed or the things you can eat. This leads to building up of temptation. You are always thinking about certain food items that you can't eat. As soon as they get a chance, they start eating in an uncontrollable manner and it leads to binge eating. It is one of the reasons people on diets gain more weight that they had lost when they went on diet.

Conclusion

Thanks for making it through to the end of this book. Let's hope it was informative and able to provide you with all of the tools you need to achieve your goals whatever they may be.

This book has been a very sincere effort in providing comprehensive information about the concept of Intermittent Fasting.

It is a concept that has garnered a lot of attention due to its amazing health benefits. However, there is still a lot of confusion about the subject in public.

People try to follow this amazing routine but are unable to get the benefits due to their inability to understand the fine things in the concept.

This book has tried to explain all the aspects of intermittent fasting so that you can reap the maximum benefits out of it.

I hope that you will be able to benefit from this book and lead a healthy and fulfilling life.

Finally, if you found this book useful in any way, a review on Amazon is always appreciated!

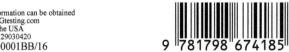